CUPPING

A Prophetical Medicine Appears in Its New Scientific Perspective

Authored by:

The great humane eminent scholar

Mohammad Amin Sheikho

(His soul has been sanctified by Al'lah)

CUPPING

A prophetical medicine appears in its new scientific perspective

Authored by:
The great humane eminent scholar
Mohammad Amin Sheikho
(His soul has been sanctified by Al'lah)

Checked and Introduced by
The Researcher and Thinker
Prof. A. K. John Alias Al-Dayrani

Copyright © Amin-sheikho.com

Our website:
www.amin-sheikho.com
info@amin-sheikho.com

Contents

CHAPTER ONE 7

The Starting Point 9

Scientific Medical Achievements of Cupping 11

Definition of Cupping 14

The History of Cupping 16

CHAPTER TWO 19

The precise scientific medical rules for cupping operation 21
First: The place of person's body for applying the cupping operation: 21
Second: The suitable age for applying cupping operation 23
Third: Timing of Applying Cupping operation 24
The seasonal time: 25

The Relation between the Moon and Cupping 29
Fourth: The Physiological Condition of the Body 32
What should the person to be cupped do on the day of Cupping? 34
The cupping operation and its psychological aspect 34

CHAPTER THREE 37

Intrigued Traditions (Hadiths) against the Cupping-Operation . 39

CHAPTER FOUR 45

We have a stance 47

CHAPTER FIVE 55

Medical Perspective in Understanding Some Mechanisms Followed by the Cupping Operation to Cure or Improve a number of Hopeless Diseases 57

- What is the role that cupping may play in spleen diseases? 57
- The effect of (cupping) on the liver. 58
- What is the effect of the (cupping) operation on immunity? .. 59
- The Effect of Cupping on the heart and the blood thrombi. 60
- The Effect of Cupping on the Digestive system? 62
- The Effect of Cupping Operation on the Nervous System, especially, the Brain. 63
- The Effect of Cupping Operation on Diabetes. 64
- The Effect of Cupping Operation on the Eye Diseases. 64
- The Effect of Cupping Operation on the Kidneys. 65
- Effect of the Cupping Operation on the Malignant Disease of the Time (Cancer) 65

CHAPTER SIX 69

The Simple Cupping Instruments 71

The Mechanism of the Cup of Cupping (Known as air-cups) 71

Application Method of the Cupping treatment 74

- Important Remarks: 76
- Remark: 77
- Important Remark 79

CHAPTER SEVEN 83

The general lab report of the systematic scientific study about the cupping operation 85

A systematic study on cupping operation, year 2000 directed by: **91**
  First: 92
  Cupping operation applied according to the correct scientific rules which are: 92
  Second: 96
  Tests on cupping operation in conditions violating its precise scientific rules: 96

Clinical medical research team **99**
  Members of the Clinical Medical Team: 99
  Members of the medical laboratory team 102

Beware of the Conjurers and of those Panting for Money! **104**

CHAPTER EIGHT 105

A Glimpse of the Life of the Eminent Scholar Mohammad Amin Sheikho **107**
  His honourable birth 107
  The sunrise of his youth & a glimpse of his deeds 108
  The stage of guidance & invitation to Al'lah 111
  A glimpse of his invitation to Al'lah, his revelation and his great guidance 112
  Joining the Highest Comrade (his death) 118

A Glimpse of the Life of the Researcher & Islamic Scholar Prof. Abdul-Kadir John alias Al-Dayrani **119**
  Prof. Abdul-Kadir said: 120

Issued to the Great Humane Eminent Scholar Mohammad Amin Sheikho (His soul has been sanctified by Al'lah) **125**

Chapter One

- **The Starting Point**
- **Scientific Medical Achievements of Cupping**
- **Definition of Cupping**
- **The History of Cupping**

The Starting Point

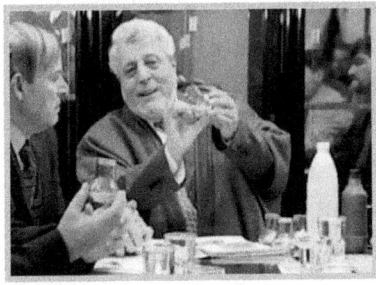

1- Prof. A. K. Al-Dayrani heading one meeting about cupping that was held with the scientific medical team supervising the research on cupping

The starting point took place when the professor and researcher A. K. John alias Al- Dayrani, began verifying and publishing the books of his great teacher, the savant Mohammad Amin Sheikho, and in fulfilling his wish in introducing the cupping operation to the human community in an authentic and scientific manner in order to enable people to get use of this marvelous medical gem.

After practically checking thousands of wondrous recovery cases during long elapsing years which culminated in the discovery of the cupping operation in its correct scientific rules.

In fact, Prof. Al-Dayrani oriented a big number of some great Syrian physicians in unique and distinct explanations about the cupping operation and its strict rules got from his teacher, the savant Mohammad Amin Sheikho.

That action on the part of prof. Al-Dayrani crystallized their opinions about the matter which encouraged them to work hand in hand with him to introduce that sublime therapeutic art to the human community which suffered for long from the grip of diseases and agonies in a scientific medical style speaking the language of the age, and taking into consideration that these precise rules were not known to anyone in the Arab world or in the western world before the great scholar M. Amin Sheikho spoke about it.

Scientific Medical Achievements of Cupping

The official broadcasting station of London (BBC), in one of its main news bulletins on 12/08/2001, declared the following:

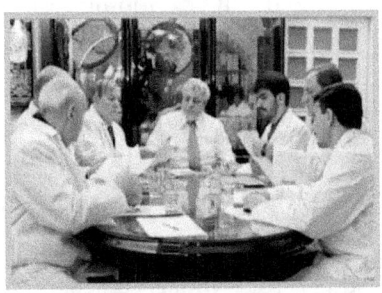

2- Prof. A. K. Al-Dayrani heading another meeting about Cupping

"The Syrians were used to betake themselves to the British capital seeking for channels of treating their diseases of which they were

desperate, or they came to make medical checkups or to perform some complicated medical operations. Such a way of acting on the part of the Syrians seemed very normal, but the unexpected act was the change in their destination from Great Britain towards the Syrian capital. A scientific medical team representing the British Royal Family began communications and dialogues with a group of Syrian physicians in Damascus in search for the cupping operation for the treatment of the hereditary disease, hemophilia. The disease confirmed its recovery in a number of sick people in Syria by means of cupping operations".

A spokesman on behalf of the prof. A. K. Dayrani, a verifier and a publisher of the books of the Damascene erudite who vitalized the cupping operation and restored its correct methods.

The added that a delegation communicated with him to acquaint themselves with the medical studies done on hundreds of Syrian and Arab patients through the precise and accurate procedures which led to astonishing results for most diseases, especially hemophilia.

He also mentioned that the first start for cupping in history was during the era of the most highborn the Messenger "Mohammad". He also added that the scientific techniques and procedures of cupping were lost as time passed until the late Damascene erudite and scholar Mohammad Amin Sheikho brought the procedures of cupping to light anew.

Dr. A. M. Al-Shalati, a specialist in neural diseases from UK and a professor in Damascus University, said to the BBC, in his talk, that the performance of cupping operations in its strict regular conditions on a group of patients gave amazing results in the complete recovery of many cases of cancer, paralysis, the problematic hemophilia, angina pectoris, Hodgkin's disease, and some improvements in asthma, rheumatism, and other cases of disease. All these cases were confirmed foundings in clinical examinations, radiological and laboratory investigations performed on patients.

§§§§§§§§§

Definition of Cupping

The word "cupping" was derived from the Arabic verbs "Hajama" and "Haj'jama" which they mean "to minimize" or "to restore to basic size", or "to diminish in volume".

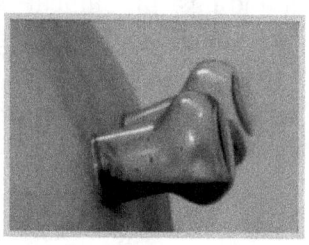

In Arabic they say, "A certain person diminished the problem", they meant that he returned the problem to its original size. There is also a verb "ahjama" which means "to withdraw or retreat from attack".

Thus he who performed the cupping operation made diseases refrain from attacking him. The increase of spoiled [1] blood in the body rendered its cessation from growing when the person became twenty-two years old, and it accumulated in the back area of the person. With advance in age, these accumulations of spoiled blood hindered the circulation of the whole blood, eventually paralyzed the work of the young red corpuscles then the body became weak and exposed to various kinds of diseases. When one performed cupping, the blood returned to its original condition and the stagnant blood went away (that blood which contained maximum rate of senile red corpuscles and their cells ghosts and

---

[1] The spoiled blood means the old red blood cells, R.B. cell ghost...

abnormal shapes of red blood cells, and other impurities).

The pressure on the blood circulation was lessened and the pure blood formed from young red corpuscles rushed to feed the cells and the body organs, and released them from harmful residues, damages and unwanted materials. Al'lah's envoy "Mohammed" (Communication with Al'lah and Peace are through him) said, "Cupping is the most helpful act for human beings to cure themselves with."

§§§§§§§§§

The History of Cupping

Cupping was old as history and it was a divine monistic norm explained by the venerated prophets and they recommended people to practice it.

Al'lah's envoy "Mohammad" (Communication with Al'lah and Peace are through him) resuscitated the procedures of cupping after being forgotten for a long time. He directed its application according to its original healthy rules.

He was so virtuous in enacting cupping for Moslems and the whole world. But on the elapse of many centuries on the passing away of the Al'lah's envoy "Mohammed" (cpth)[2] , the rules of cupping were gradually forgotten due to negligence, dereliction and abstention until those rules were obliterated and lost.

There were certainly some sinful hands that put much lies in it and its basics until people abstained from using it and forgot it completely. It was true that few people practiced it, but unluckily they did not get use of it, or they did not get healthy benefit of it at all until people disclaimed it for they did not get its promising benefit.

People used to perform cupping in winter and summer, or after physical toil and fatigue, or after breakfast though it must be applied before breakfast. But eventually, the late humane savant, Mohammad Amin

---

[2] (Communication with Al'lah and Peace are through him)

Sheikho revived the norm (Sunnah) in its precise rules which were mentioned in his book.

He revealed its rules and put them in their exact place on the human body for application. He also put forth the general secret of its healing mechanism which said "to rid one's self of impure blood". He returned this medical therapeutic art to its effective scientific role and disclosed its rules and principles to his acquaintances, relatives and friends. In turn, they informed their acquaintances, relatives, friends and neighbors and all the people until it spread in many countries and even all people.

When people gained great healthy physical, psychological and feasible benefits, they increased in number in using it during the last years. They realized marvels in curing incurable diseases[3] of the era as cancer, paralysis, angina pectoris, hemophilia, migraine, and the like.

§§§§§§§§

---

[3] diseases can't be cured by recent Medicine

Chapter Two

- **The precise scientific medical rules for cupping operation**
- **The Relation between the Moon and Cupping**

The precise scientific medical rules for cupping operation

"Discovered by the Savant M. Amin Sheikho"

The Precise scientific medical rules, elucidated by the savant M. Amin Sheikho in his book which the medical team has used in its scientific research work, can be summarized as follows:

- First: The place of body for applying the cupping operation.

- Second: The suitable age for cupping operation

- Third: Time of the cupping operation

- Fourth: The physiological situation of the body.

§§§§§§§§§

First: The place of person's body for applying the cupping operation:

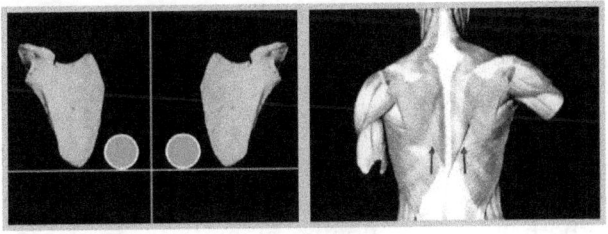

3- The place of body for applying the cupping operation

It is: near the lower end of the shoulder blade (the scapula) in the two symmetric locations between the spine and the inside limit of the scapula.

The cupping operation makes a kind of blood congestion in the upper part of the back "these two symmetric places of back" by using (air cups). This cup is applied on the upper frontal part of the back, near the lower end of the scapulae and on the two sides of the spine.

This is because it is the calmest area in the body and void of moving joints. This area is a net of plexus capillaries of much ramification and profusion which makes the flow rate of blood circulation much less where the blood of the body precipitates its harmful precipitations (such as cell ghosts and dead of red blood cells ...) in it.

We made a lab study on this case, we found that the white corpuscles were less in this area of the back on the other hand the cupping blood (the withdrawn blood by cupping) was full of cell ghosts, dead and abnormal red blood cells which made the cupping operation very suitable here. We per-formed cupping operations in places on the leg, the two jugular veins, and the back near the pelvis. The cupping blood in these places was similar to the vein blood.

Second: The suitable age for applying cupping operation

Concerning men:

It is incumbent upon every male who reaches the twenty-two years of age to undergo cupping operation from the seventeenth day of the lunar month which comes in the spring season of every year until the twenty-seventh day of it.

Childhood and adulthood stages require big quantities of iron because the body is in the phase of growth. These quantities are not completely supplied by food for this growing body. This decrease in iron is equalized by the way of digesting the senile and spoiled red blood cells in the liver and the spleen, and the phagocytes of the body forming the stored iron reserve which are kept for the body needs.

The body in general and its bone marrow in particular benefit from these red blood cells after transforming them suitably in a series of operations "metabolism" producing the iron (hemo) and amino acids (globin) which are used by the growing body to supply its need of iron in addition to reconstruction of new red generations of red blood cells . After the twenty years, the big consumption of the spoiled red blood cells stops for the cessation of body's growth. So the surplus of them become big and "they must be discharged".

Concerning the women:

It is incumbent upon every female who passes the menopause stage.

The woman has a natural outlet through which she can release herself from bad blood. During menstruation period, her blood circulation becomes at the apex of activity. When woman reaches her menopause stage, her menses ceases and she becomes subject to the same conditions of man who reaches the age of twenty- two.

Thus she enters a new physiological phase leading to psychological and physical changes paving the way to the rise of various diseases such as high blood pressure, coronary insufficiency and diabetes, and the like. In this situation, cupping becomes inevitable and there is no other alternative for it.

It makes woman returns to her normal psychological and physical case. If she refuses to perform the simple cupping operation, her body becomes a pasture for maladies and prone to diseases.

§§§§§§§§

Third: Timing of Applying Cupping operation

To Apply Cupping operation you have to consider four appointed times:

The annual time:

The Messenger (cpth) said: **"How good the wont in cupping is!"**

Thus, it is usually performed from year to year for both the healthy and the patient. It is a prophylaxis for the healthy and a medicine (treatment) and a protection (prophylaxis) for the patient.

The seasonal time:

The Messenger (cpth) said, **"Relieve yourselves from the intensity of heat by cupping."**

Therefore cupping must be performed before the summer season because heat is most intense at this time of the year. Hence the best season is the spring.

Cupping must be performed every year in the spring season, namely in April and May (In Syria and other countries around it).

Before giving the scientific interpretation of this appointed time (its physiological effect on our bodies), we must give a simple glimpse about the function of the blood in regulating the animal heat.

As it is known water constitutes the maximum proportion in the blood, (90%) of its plasma. Since water has basic properties that differentiate it from other liquids known in nature, these properties make water the best assistant liquid to help regulating the animal heat in a living being. This property has a high faculty of storing heat than any other liquid or solid material. Therefore it stores the heat it receives in its passage through the more active and warm tissues and carries it to other tissues of less warmth in its movement through the various parts of the body. Therefore blood has (the proportion of water in its formation and its round trip in the tissues of the body) a high faculty in transmitting heat higher than any other faculty of various tissues in the body. Therefore blood is the first recipient and the first main influenced tissue by the outside heat (of all the body tissues) which is effective on the body. It sucks heat from the body tissues to transport it to the less warm ones, and vice versa it sucks coolness from the body tissues to transport it to the warm ones.

In view of the continuous blood circulation, it acts in regulating the animal heat by warming the cool parts or cooling the warm parts until the animal heat remains constant. The chance for cupping is realized two times in the year, i.e. in April and in May, and perhaps a third time in late of March if the warmth comes at the end of it with only the decrease of the crescent.

In this time of the spring, we trace the lunar month until it becomes the 17th day of it, and then one can undergo cupping operation in one of these days (from the seventeenth day until the twenty-seven day inclusive).

If he misses the first month, the advent of the (17th) of the next lunar month (in which cupping is permissible), he can also make up for the chance. Naturally, there are some irregular years when April is also intensive in chilliness, then we must wait until May, or we could perhaps perform the cupping operation in April.

If the (17) of the lunar month in April has cold weather, we wait until the weather becomes moderate and warm during the period of this lunar month (17-27) then we start cupping. Therefore, the matter is limited by the general rule which we cannot overcome for it is springtime (April, May and perhaps late of March and the early of June) from the seventeenth day until the twenty-seventh day of the lunar month exclusively depending on the rise in temperature in March and the drop of it at the beginning of June if both changes occur along with the decrease of the lunar month. In this way, we get use of one-third of the year to perform the cupping operation.

The Monthly Time:

The Messenger of God (cpth) said, **"Cupping is most detestable at the beginning of the crescent, but it is curing when the full moon begins to decrease."**

Therefore, we must follow up the recommendation of the Messenger (cpth) on the lunar month when the time of the annual cupping comes (springtime in its two months, April and May).

For example, when April comes we follow up the progression of the lunar month which comes in this month (April), and when the seventeenth day of the lunar month comes, it will certainly be the first day for performing Cupping. Therefore, cupping starts from the seventeenth day (inclusive) until the twenty-seventh day (inclusive).

§§§§§§§§

The Relation between the Moon and Cupping

What secret it was that made the Messenger (cpth) apprise of the time of cupping to be in the springtide with the progression of the lunar month from only the seventeenth day until the twenty-seventh day of it!

We know that the moon has a pull effect on the earth despite its little diameter (3478 km), and its mass constitutes one part out of (80) parts of the mass of the earth, and the distance of it from the earth is a distance of (385.000 km), this short distance makes its pulling force have a great influence on the oceans where they rise to form the tide, even the earth's crust is never free from these effects.

The crust of the North American continent heaves up to fifteen centimeters when the moon interposes its sky. The moon has also another effect which helps sap to rise in its circulation in the high trees.

The two French professors (Jubet and Galieh de Fond) noticed that the moon has an effect on animals from its birth as a crescent until it becomes a full-moon. The sexual activates increase gradually in animals, poultry and birds.

They also noticed that poultry give more eggs in this period more than the period of senility when the moon begins its gradual atrophy to hunchback phase, then to the last lunar quarter, and to waning. According to special notice, it is found that there is a period of activity and much energy in animals connected with the lunar stages. They also noticed that poultry and some domesticated animals, and fishes, animals and lobsters of the Indian Ocean and the Red Sea produce more eggs in certain periods of the moon faces.

The moon reaches the climax of its effect when it is full-moon. It affects blood pressure producing higher level of pressure and in stimulating the blood circulation, so the sexual craving is excited. Also some western countries suffer much from the increase in the rate of crimes and assaults in nights and days of the full-moon.

During the first days of the lunar month, i.e. from the first day until the fifteenth, blood-flow is stimulated and it reaches its maximal limit and eventually it pokes all the blood residues and impurities which precipitated along the walls of the deep and superficial and in all the ramifications of the blood vessels in the tissues (exactly as, in turn, it - as a big spoon- stirs the water of the seas so as the salts in them don't precipitate). Likewise, when the moon begins to decrease from (17 – 27), the blood can carry these residues and impurities to the calmest parts of the body where they settle in the shoulder blades area.

The tide of the seas due to the lunar pull begins to weaken from 17 to 27 of the lunar calendar. Since the cupping operation is performed in the morning after sleep and rest for the body and the blood circulation, and the moon is still rising despite the sunrise in the morning. The moon will have a little tidal effect during the performance of cupping. This situation is very good for our work for the moon still has the effect of pulling the blood from inside to the outside (the inner blood of the peripheral blood and the peripheral blood surrounding the opening of the cup). This situation has an excellent effect in performing a successful and profitable cupping operation to release the body from its impure blood.

If the cupping operation is performed in the middle of the lunar days (12-13-14-15), the strong pull of the moon stimulates the blood, and the blood will lose much of its young corpuscles, the Merciful God does not wish that for His servant-mankind. But the first days of the moon (crescent) do not let it do its job in carrying the blood residues and impurities from the inside to the outside in order to gather in the upper part of the back as it has been mentioned before.

§§§§§§§§§

The Daily Time:
The cupping operation is usually performed in the early morning after the sunrise, but the time of stopping it in each day is pointed according to the heat level of the weather. If the weather stills moderate during the day,

we continue applying it until noon; such timing is permissible but not desirable.

It is better for cupping to be performed at the first hours of the day (because cupping must be performed while the person is still without having breakfast).

If a person remains without having breakfast for late hours of the day, he becomes tired and dizzy for the delay of having his breakfast and having performed the cupping operation. In order to avoid all these problems and to perform a correct useful cupping operation, we must hasten to perform it in the early hours of the day from seven o'clock till ten o'clock, and in a needful situation when the time is the last day (27 of the lunar calendar) of performing it and the weather is still moderate and not intense in heat, in this case you can perform the operation until eleven o'clock or more before the noon. When we delay the operation until (midday), we certainly walk, move and work.

This motivates the blood circulation a little and scoops with it the harmful precipitations (such as cell ghosts and dead red blood cells ...) which temporary precipitate under the shoulder blades, eventually the benefit from cupping is not complete.

Fourth: The Physiological Condition of the Body

The cupping operation must be done before the breakfast. The Messenger of God (cpth) said,

"Cupping before breakfast is optimal, and it has cure and benediction."

It is forbidden for a person to be cupped to take in any morsel whatsoever in the morning of cupping, but to remain fasting until it is performed upon him. He is permitted to drink a cup of coffee or tea for the sugar it contains is little and it does not need complicated digestive operations which stir the blood, activate the blood circulation, affect the blood pressure, and the heart beats. Also this little quantity of tea or coffee contains a simple nerve stimulant which makes the person undergo cupping in a wakeful case.

For this reason the Prophet (cpth) prohibited eating before applying cupping for it activates the digestive system and the blood circulation in order to recompense the digestive operations which lead to the increase in heart beats, blood flow, and a high blood pressure. This case will move the precipitated residues of the sluggish and retired blood in the superficial and deep blood vessels and capillaries in the region of the upper back (these unwanted materials of blood gather during sleeping). Also blood flow is activated during the distribution of the digested nutrients in order to feed the body tissues. Such a situation does not fit cupping.

If cupping is performed in similar condition, the blood isn't filtered by this operation (Cupping), so the withdrawn blood is the working blood (not the spoiled blood which is full of impurities as dead red blood cells and R.B. cell ghosts …) and we have lost the expected benefit from cupping. In this case, the cupped person will also suffer from slight vertigo or syncope as a result of the insufficient quantity of blood which irrigates the brain.

What should the person to be cupped do on the day of Cupping?

The person to be cupped can eat a kind of food that is easy for digestion such as vegetables, fruits and candies. It is usually offered to the cupped-person a dish of vegetable salad mixed with bits of toasted bread, and sprayed with olive oil and vinegar.

The dish is known by the name of (Fat'toosh) known to the Damascenes; and a dish of olives may be added to the meal.

The cupping operation and its psychological aspect

The Damascene erudite Mohammad Amin Sheikho explained this point by saying: "Cupping is the prophets' advice". For the whole fact, and in implementing this wholesome therapeutic art, which was recommended for application by the most honored prophets such as our masters Moses, Jesus and Mohammed (cptt)[4], and their followers as the savant

---

[4] (Communication with Al'lah and Peace are through them)

Mohammad Amin Sheikho, the soul of the cupped-person tends to follow up those great physicians, the Physicians of the heart (soul), the inclination of the cupped-person's soul towards them while their insights are staring incessantly at the Almighty Curing God, and there is no cure except Him, this inclination makes his soul immersed in the Almighty's Light, therefore the cupped-person's soul is cured by the Godly Light forwarded on the prophets.

Yes, cupping cures psychic ailments and ignoble characteristics and changes them into the properties of perfection. And because of detestable statuses, and before performing cupping, the cupped-person may have contracted some diseases so as that his heart is to be cured by resorting himself to God in order to attain the recovery. Since he has followed the teachings of God as iterated by His Most Honorable Messenger; and his soul has directed itself unconsciously to its Creator. His soul has improved and his heart has eavesdropped to the teachings of God.

After that there is no need for a disease that may protect him from the evils of his spirit and of the acts for his heart has become virtuous.

If the heart is reformed, the whole body becomes immuned against diseases. This psychological advantage has a great effect on recovery according to the tendency towards God. If it is strong, the cupped-person is acquitted of all diseases, and all diseases abstain protectively from attacking him.

If the tendency towards God is feeble, the improvement is relative, but the benefit must be realized whatsoever.

Cupping is all helpful. There is no harm at all in applying it. And I think the experiments on cupping for the elapsed century is enough to approve; there is no resulting harm to any person at all from applying it according to its precise rules.

Former experiments are the best proof for certainty.

§§§§§§§§

Chapter Three

- **Intrigued Traditions (Hadiths) against the Cupping-Operation**

Intrigued Traditions (Hadiths) against the Cupping-Operation

A certain person may say: "I have read some of the prophetic traditions[5] which prevent cupping on days of Saturday, Sunday, Wednesday, Friday, Tuesday, and Thursday, and I have found that there is contradiction in them. Some of these traditions prefer cupping to be performed, and others prohibit doing it. Which Hadith is the right one? Rightness is whole in one and it is never pluralized!"

In answer to this inquiry, we say: that all the prophetic traditions are correct and strong and there is not any weak one among them at all. How could weakness sneak to them, and the Almighty God has witnessed in describing the Prophet in The Holy Qur'an, An-Najm Fortress, Verse (3): **"Nor does he speak of (his own) desire."** If contradictory is found between a certain tradition and the Noble Qur'an, and this denotes that there is doubt about its credibility and its fallacy is most clear, and the Messenger of God is exonerated from it, he didn't speak it at all. There are many traditions that were forged and foisted in order to let people run in confusion and divert themselves from reality and fall preys in labyrinth. But no one can divert himself from rightness and reality except that one who has neglected

---

[5] Sayings are belonged to the prophet Mohammed (cpth) by spiteful persons, but actually he (cpth) didn't say them.

his mind and does not give research its rightness which is attained thorough examination and comparison according to the Holy Book "Qur'an", logic and rightness. However, he who uses his mind contemplating in the wonders of the universe and thinking about his end in this life and his future in the hereafter.

Then, he attains the real faith, that changes the disbeliever to a savant after his insight is opened, and the wax of his ears vanishes, and the haze of his eyes disappears, and his spirit "heart" have been purified, and becomes perfect after he has loved and adored the people of perfection, and the Messenger of God (cpth) who is the Master of Perfection and high moralities, He becomes by this divine trustworthy bond, which has no schism, able to put the proof against himself and against the others, depending on what he has known and understood from the Holy Book "Qur'an" which becomes his reference, his support and his scale (He who grasps it in practical life saves himself, and he who leaves it to other ones (books) perishes himself.

Therefore, through the real faith alone man can distinguish between the exact tradition and the fabricated one. If the utterance is contradictory and different, that means the tradition is concocted by people, and not said by the prophet.

God said, **"Certainly, you have different ideas. Turned aside there from is he who is turned aside."**

The Holy Qur'an,
Fortress (51) Adh-Dharyat (8 - 9)

Whereas the rightful utterance which is approved by the Book of God is harmonious to a high level of harmony by the right logic and irrefutable evidence, so we find in it the uprightness and integrity of humanity.

The Messenger who has adhered himself to God in such a way that he has surpassed the whole world and all people in understanding the Book of the Almighty Al'lah.

Almighty Al'lah says in Holy Qur'an Ar-Ra'd Fortress (43):

"And those disbelievers say:" You are not a Messenger. "O. Mohammed Say: It is Sufficient That God is the witness who is the right path "me or you". And who has the knowledge of the holy Book like me?" And who could understand it like me? Such was his reply to the deniers of his messages and of his prophecy and the skeptical persons in his calling.

As well as, those who have sincerely followed him, getting true insight, will never be deceived by the ornament of utterance and its vanity.

The Almighty Al'lah Says: **"O. Mohammed, say; this is my way, I invite unto Allah with sure knowledge, I and whosoever follows me...."**

The Holy Qur'an,
Fortress (12) Yusuf (108)

As for those narrated traditions, which permit performing cupping on days of Monday, Tuesday and Thursday; and forbids its performance on days of Wednesday, Saturday and Sunday, were weakened by Alhafez Ibn Hijr in Alfat'h (the Conquest) (12/256), and the late Imam Almajlisi showed their contradictions.

We shall, for exclusive example, bring a pattern for you and leave the verdict to you, my dear brother reader.

The first tradition: from Ibn Omar "may God be pleased with him" said, **"Apply cupping treatment on Thursday..."**[6]

The second tradition: **"Never be cupped on Thursday. He, who has been performed on, misfortune, affects him..."**[7]

Today, there are so many contradictory traditions which tell you to be cupped on Tuesday, and others tell you not to be cupped on such a day.

---

[6] (Ibn Majah /3487/).
[7] Kanz Al-Ummal (workmen's treasure) /Hindi/ (28158).

This contradiction denotes to their falseness and incredibility, and aims at confusion and liquefaction of the traditions of the favorite Prophet about cupping.

All these are prejudiced intrigues whereas the rightful one is the one which the clear logic accepts it through the practical fact, and that which you find it aligns with the tradition of the Messenger of God, that does not confine cupping on days of Saturday, or Sunday, or Monday, or Tuesday…etc. but it defines the cupping time according to the lunar month, from his saying: " **Cupping is detested at the beginning of the crescent, and it is not hoped for benefit until the crescent decreases**".

It was told by Al-Hindi in his Kanz Al-Ummal (28113), by al-Ajlouni in 'Kashf Al-khafa' (Uncovering of the concealment), and by Ibn Al-Jawzi in Tathkarat Almawdhooaat /207/ (Memo of subjects).

This tradition was backed by another one in his saying: **"The best days for you to be cupped are the seventeenth day, the nineteenth day, and the twenty-first day (of the lunar month)"**[8]

This honored tradition denotes the incredibility of the traditions which prohibit most days of the week: Saturday, Sunday, Wednesday, Thursday, Friday, and

---

[8] Sunan Ibn Majah, Al-tib, No./3469/(Norms of Medicine).

Tuesday … for a clear reason you yourself can discover it.

Let us suppose that the seventeenth day of the lunar month comes on Friday and this means that the nineteenth day of it will surely be Sunday, and the twenty-first day of it will be Tuesday.

Let us also suppose that the seventeenth day comes on Thursday, then the nineteenth will be Saturday, and the twenty-first will be Monday… and so on.

The inconstancy of the days in relation with the dates of the lunar month because the lunar month is changing from month to another, and from year to year.

This proves the abrogation of the traditions and of the claims that prohibit applying cupping on some days despite they are in a true time of performing cupping as they are in the spring time and after the decreasing of crescent …, and it confirms the futility of such traditions in a clear way.

The Prophet (cpth) is innocent of such fabrications

And praise belongs to God at the beginning and at the end

§§§§§§§§

Chapter Four

- **We have a stance**

We have a stance

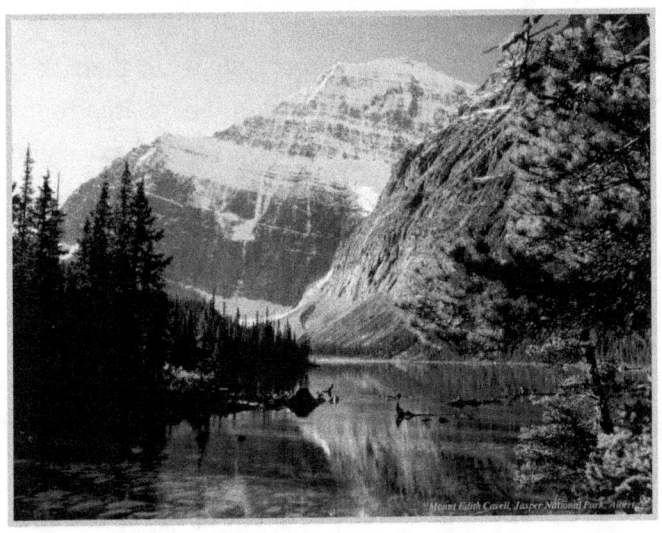

You have the right to be astonished and to wonder at the secrets of life, new for new, and to implement the tradition of the Messenger of God, "Quest for knowledge from the cradle to the grave" He also request you to meditate on your origin until your end in the grave, i.e. by thinking of death so that your soul fears this end, then it resorts to God in order to see the indisputable facts by means of the light of the Almighty God even if you have passed your age, however it extends, and you have pierced the times roaming in the horizons and oceans of sciences, which do not come to end. Your sight is inverted myopically; and your knowledge has bequeathed you the secrets of life in prostration to that solemnity, and the mysterious and obvious Divine Greatness in diversities of its creation which were found in unprecedented example.

There are groups of great cosmic systems in their very strong constructions running in orbits. There are groups of stars staggering in wonderful majesty and ravishing beauty.

Who is the one that made these mighty powers which emit light in spite of their distances, and cosmic forces in cohesive connection and disconnection in such a way as the solidity of building stones decorating the sky? The earth is subjected to their forces, day and night. Some clear ones of them are guides to travelers in deep seas or vast arid lands. Some of them have clandestine effect on the seas that prevent them from scattering and flowing away. Hence, the moon is but a spherical stony mass revolving in its sky that it (the moon) cannot exceeds its orbit.

It in order and uniformity rises slowly, looks down with its beautiful face arousing the hiding places of the seas to keep corruption away as it arouses the blood in the bodies on the first moonlit nights to remove from them all spoiled blood by cupping.

The earth in its revolution covers years and epochs without tiredness or weariness. The mountains are unshakable above it regulating its revolution and preventing its swaying. God said, "And He has affixed into the Earth Mountains standing firm, lest it should shake with you, and rivers and roads that you may guide yourselves."

*The Holy Qur'an,
Fortress (15) An-Nahl (15)*

The revolving of the earth originates the night and the day following each other in increasing and decreasing until everything gives out its fruit in a management of wonderful regulation, as a result, the four seasons are created where the victuals become of various kinds after watering the thirsty land, preparing the fields for work, and flowering of trees to bear for you the big delicacies and nourishments and the small ones as vitamins in the form of cordiality and gifts as a great pledge for you, O. Man.

Who has created all? And who has innovated all? And who is the regulator of forces? Who makes the earth revolving and brings the night followed by the day? Who sends rain…? Did all these inanimate things exist themselves by themselves? And did they organize themselves by themselves? And who provides the planets, the sun, the moon and the galaxies with light? Is the blind subjected Nature which created the eyesights and the endowed by eyesight? Or there is a great controlling creating potency that has created, innovated and originated!

What about the glaciers lying down in its two poles? And what will make you know what it is?

They are one of the secrets of existence. The high property of man lies down in them excepting all other creatures. Outpouring and very clear water comes to us without harm, or effort or toil. It is like Al-fijeh water of Damascus which we enjoy clear, healthy, cool, fresh and abundant in bliss in summer or winter.

All germs in the earth which work, insects, animals, and fishes in the seas, all of these various kinds in their life and work are working together and collaborating under our control and disposition of the human beings.

What about the human body and what do we know about it?

It is another sea. It is one of the seas of the universe. Diving into it and delving into its secrets would be a kind of miracle of the time. It makes man fall prostrated to the greatness of its builder and founder. The human science is still at its early daybreak of exploring and verfying this sea "the human body" in spite of the high technological advance.

Yes! Let us travel every day to the shiny hands of God while doing miracles in these cosmos, in the mountains, the sea, and in the sky "And also in your own selves. Will you not see"

The Holy Qur'an,
Fortress (51) Adh-Dharyat (21)

Let us kneel before this great hand hoping that the luminous water of real life may penetrate into our thirsty hearts, in order to be infatuated with Him the Almighty, to be free from these materialistic screens that stand between us and Him and His the Almighty Love. Then we may have the high state of reverence for Him, and return to the instinct of perfection in order to save ourselves from the eternal loss. Our energies are deposited in our trust, and this deposit is temporal, it will not last forever. Tomorrow, we shall be without sight, hearing, smelling, willing, air, water, sunlight, or moonlight; and we shall be without brothers or friends where aspirations decline and we lose hope in a ditch in the ground "the grave" which made a reward for our pursuit and panting after this world without penetration through it to its most High Maker. For these reasons and for His love, mercy for us, God, the Almighty, knows all that, and after having varied His bounties and graces, He made us look at loss and extinction, and since we are rational and our religion is logical He elevated us by His Prophet (cpth) by what He conferred upon him (cpth) the sciences, secrets and miracles of this world, and the science of the true psychiatry. So he "the prophet (cpth)" unveiled to us some secrets of the spirit saying; man is always with whom he loves. So, if any one adheres himself to something or somebody other than God, he is cut off. Everything happening in the universe is passing to extinction except God.

He who loves God an authentic love which poured out from deep thinking, he who glorifies and becomes righteous for fear of losing the affection of the Beloved the Almighty (Glory be unto Him), and expels his heart from the love of villainous world before the coming of death. Then death will be his masterpiece, and the Day of Resurrection will be the day of eternal hilarity for him. But he who has abandoned God and starts enjoying himself in the vanities of the world; and he has not made of it a mount for his high advent to his God by doing good and charity. But he remained stumbling in directing its devilish fancies and contents as if he were a toy in satanic hands without knowing and this is a sheer misery and a great loss.

Whereas that great thinker, our exemplar (cpth), searched for the owner of this universe.

He believed in God frequently from a new starting point, from the marvels of the great universe, he found the way to God is open in every time, day and night, from here until doomsday, to the eternity of the eternals.

Let us try to escape from the snare of loving of the embittering world even if we could remember for a while death and its horrors so as to fear the destiny. We shall then throw away the despicable world from our hearts, and we could head ourselves to the Great God, and keep our contemplation concentrated on his benefactions as a daily supply in the morning and at sunset between the friends and the beloved ones in gardens and on roads in the summer and the winter hoping that the autumn of our life will turn into springtide, and our faces will lighten by the lightning of the gleams of the faith in God.

Then we may perceive this eulogy to find ourselves glorifying God through His make during our vigilance and our sleep then our graves will be one of the orchards of paradise by improvement and uprightness of our faith and acts with a Mighty King. And for that let the rivals compete.

Chapter Five

- **Medical Perspective in Understanding Some Mechanisms Followed by the Cupping Operation to Cure or Improve a number of Hopeless Diseases**

Medical Perspective in Understanding Some Mechanisms Followed by the Cupping Operation to Cure or Improve a number of Hopeless Diseases

What is the role that cupping may play in spleen diseases?

Splenomegalies may be due to the need of increasing the splenic work. For example, some reasons which causes these Splenomegalies are;

Infectious inflammatory causes: It is believed that this kind of Splenomegaly caused by infectious inflammatory factor results from the increasing in spleen's defensive activity, or due to the increasing need to refine certain compounds from the blood.

And the congestive causes: this kind of Splenomegaly caused by the congestive causes results from the increase in pressure in portal circulation or in the general blood circulation.

The amplification may also be due to over productivity of reticals-endothelia cells for the spleen to withdraw the spoiled cells from the blood, or due to the myeloid metaplasia, or the amplification may be due to blood rubeosis, or infiltration lesion where the spleenphagias are filled with spoiled materials which accumulated due to the effect of these diseases.

We have found in this respect that the cupping operation is a must solution for such cases (Splenomegalies). Moreover, cupping can stimulate the reticuloendothelial cells to carry out its important immunity role against germs, parasites, fungi and protozoons.

It is clear that cupping application according to its rules is a secondary spleen which forms a main assistant for the spleen in the blood filtration from all unwanted materials and spoiled and dead blood cells. So cupping Medicine is a very important protective of, and curing treatment in such cases of spleen problems.

The effect of (cupping) on the liver.

When cupping removes the spoiled and senile corpuscles and the impurities from the blood, and it increases blood flow in all tissues and organs, consequently in the liver tissue. So, the liver cells will be activated and then the whole liver will be activated to perform its other functions in a complete performing. It will transform the cholesterol and the excessive triglycerides by its metabolic function, and stores the excessive sugar in blood with help from the pancreas in reducing glucose level to normal one in the diabetics. And the liver will be more active in rescuing the body from poisons, this activate all its systems including the brain and nervous system so the general health of body is better.

it also heightens the regeneration of spoiled tissues in the body because the liver is responsible for the production of the necessary protein for continuation of life and growth, it is clear that cupping medicine is a cure or main improving of all hepatic problems including all types of hepatitis, and prevents from or curing the hypertension of the portal vein and all resulting dangerous problems.

Prof. Dr. A. G. Jabakji, the specialist in neuro-microscopic surgery from Holland, says, "The implementation of cupping as it has been recommended is an explicit and clear entrance to complete health and good recovery. It supplies man with great power and energy by way of opening and cleaning the fine blood vessels within which blood precipitates and forms residues on its walls, and such a case is one of the causes of migraine, heart and liver diseases, and other ailments of the age."

If we consider the hepatic Enzymes as a criterion for all treated cases where the levels of them are high, the findings are; after cupping they return to their normal levels.

What is the effect of the (cupping) operation on immunity?

The cupping operation increases the ability and activity of the immunity system due to the increased activity of the reticals-endothelial system, and the good blood flow through the tissues and organs heightens the immunity of the body because that the pathogens in the body are more subjected to the immunity system unites.

Interferon is the quickest defensive line to be formed and secreted after the exposure of the body to any virus. Prof. Kanteel says, "That the leukocytes can produce interferon in a rate exceeding ten times what the other body cells produce." The tests of cupping blood showed a presence of very slight rate of leukocytes in it in addition to its great effect in producing the immunity defensive cells as the phagocytes which destroy pathogenic agents. this development in the stem (initial) blood cells go toward leukocytes formation, that the case of body demanding increasing in white blood cells in order to defend the body against the pathogenic agents. Here we can say: cupping keeps the leukocytes (there is just a very slight rate of leukocytes in cupping blood) and activates its production that helps in producing interferon in abundant quantities to face the hepatic virus or cancer cells.

This is what we have seen through the tests which the lab team has performed.

The Effect of Cupping on the heart and the blood thrombi.

In this era we hear every day about a sudden death and paralysis. These incidents are attributed to blood clots which are nothing but an agglomeration of red and white corpuscles, platelets and fibrin fibers crowded together at the ramifications of arteries to form a clot, its main happening is hypertension. The cupping operation has a great preventive role as it was mentioned in some of Hadiths that it prevents (hyperemia).

In the dictionary of "Lissan Al-Arab" hyperemia means "agitation and increase," This description applies also on arterial hypertension and real increase in red corpuscles (poly Cythemia vera; Erythremia).

The disturbance of the cardiac system may be caused by ischemia or oxyachrestia. Also myocardia infarction is due to ischemia resulting from arterial stenosis (arteriosclerosis) and the thrombi themselves when they are in these coronary arteries.

The angina pectoris is generated when there is a decrease in supplying the heart tissue with the necessary Oxygen. Because the fat precipitations have partly blocked up the coronary artery. Then the high level of arterial hypertension may lead to complications such as: cardiac insufficiency, angina pectoris and encephala vascular incident. The long arterial hypertension may cause heart enlargement, and atherosclerosis.

So, applying cupping is the best solution to prevent and treat such cases, as cupping decreases the level of fat (triglyceride, cholesterol) in blood to normal one, gets rid of hypertension and increases the blood flow through heart tissue after cleaning the arteries and preventing them from atherosclerosis.

The Effect of Cupping on the Digestive system?

The blood stagnation in the veins of the stomach and the intestines destroys their secretive and absorption functions and that will lead to severe bleeding, especially the vessels of the stomach, the intestines, the esophagus and the rectum, and blood clots in the legs and feet, hemorrhoids, and severe menstruation "in women", all of what mentioned above leads blood pressure to go down.

So, cupping medicine activates the blood flow and consequently prevents blood from congestion in the digestive system. Therefore cupping prevents and treats all the above mentioned cases.

Most problems with hemorrhoids which patients come to an end after performing cupping. The heightening blood pressure with a sluggish blood circulation leads to harm the biliary tracts and increase the density of the bile. Here cholesterol and bilirubin start to crystallize and that hinders the circulation of the arterial blood.

Whereas the compactness of the aged red corpuscles and their precipitation result in the impeded circulation in portal vein. Eventually, the tension of the portal vein heightens to push a part of the blood to the peripheral circulation round the liver through vessels anastomosis, consequently the spleen congests and enlarges and also does the venous vessels in the pancreas leading to its atrophy and its inability to do its functions. This is what we have seen.

In fact, the cupping operation is a prevention and cure for all these problems and saves us from the trouble.

The Effect of Cupping Operation on the Nervous System, especially, the Brain.

The vascular incidents of the brain can be referred to two things:

• The ischemia and its rate (80%).

• Bleeding and its rate (20%).

If the ischemia extends, it will lead to brain congestion and results in hemiplegia. And this is what we have avoided its occurrence by performing a cupping operation.

The cupping operation is helpful in regulating the blood coming to the brain. It is also found to be useful in cases of memory weakness and lack of concentration. It also helps in controlling and regulating feelings and affections. .

Cupping was also mentioned for its usefulness for epilepsy and in improving the hearing if the cause was ischemia, and the stability resulting from lack of the coming blood.

The Effect of Cupping Operation on Diabetes.

One of the factors of heightening the rate of sugar in blood is ischemic the case where the body is stimulated to liberate glucose in order to raise the activity of its organs.

Unluckily, the cause is not in the burning or in the ability, but the ischemic meager. And this explains the secret of immediate recovery for diabetic people soon after performing the operation. The activity of the liver and pancreas share much in reducing the level of sugar in the blood. This is what we have seen while performing the operation.

The Effect of Cupping Operation on the Eye Diseases.

Cupping, while playing its role in removing from the blood all that impedes its movement and prevents it from stagnation. In this way, it activates the blood circulation and improves the perfusion of tissues and organs, and at the same time, it raises the activities of the various organs and systems of the body in addition to what result from the re-arrangement of the hormone secretion leading to raise the immunity and defense of the body and its systems, especially the brain, the optic nerve, and the retina improving, in this way, the general state of the eyesight.

The Effect of Cupping Operation on the Kidneys.

The two kidneys usually do their duty of cleaning the body from nitrogen products, regulate the concentration of sodium, and metabolize the body liquids. They also concentrate the ions in blood and the balance of PH in the body, the deficiency of blood perfusion to the kidneys breaks down the kidneys from doing their elimination function and that may cause kidney failure, or to fall victim of Boliva disease which affects the brain and kills its cells. Cupping eliminates the ischemia from the kidneys and encourages them to function their duties to the best and that will increase the resistance of the body against diseases in general.

Effect of the Cupping Operation on the Malignant Disease of the Time (Cancer)

The accumulation of blood impurities will affect negatively the flow of blood, the perfusion of the tissues and organs will decrease, then the heart will exert more effort to secure their requirements. When the outpouring of blood lessens from the liver, the blood impurities deviates it from its most important duty in removing poisonous materials. The function of the spleen will be lowered in its immunity level in producing antibodies and in straining the blood from strange elements. The work of the systems will recede little by little. The person will not immediately feel these changes in his body until old age when situations become worse, the troubles appear, and diseases creep upon him.

For this reason we find that the rate of infection in cancer is greater in aged people than it is in others. All this is due to the absence of cupping. When the outside factors, such as chemical and radiological elements, and psychological impacts, the body becomes a prey for these aggressors.

This is not all, for the body cells proliferated madly until they revolted against this body, and it was cancer. Any disturbance in the systems of the body leads to disturbance in the hormone disequilibrium with the outside factors. But the result was bigger than a weak immunity system weakened by ischemia. The organism recognizes the cancerous cells and considers them strange and forms antibodies against them seeking to control this tumor and trying to stop its diffusion, and the tumor appears when the equilibrium tends to the advantage of the cancerous cells.

Cancer has grown up when its cells overcome the immunity system, and the immunity system is linked with the systems and organs of the body, and the whole forms an integrated unity.

If the liver worked in a high competence and saved the body from poisons, and stored, analyzed and combined, and the spleen accomplished its turn by changing its immunity cells, the T-B phagocytes, into secreting cells for globulins, and the humeral immunity was strengthened, and the two kidneys were purifying and organizing the mineral salts in a high efficiency as the other systems and organs of the body do, then the body will restrain all outside effects and remains safe and sound. Statistics have shown that people, who took medicines to inhibit immunity when they performed renal transplantation operations, were more exposed to infection by cancerous tumors than normal ones in a rate that reaches (35) times more. Some cases were found in the Americans that (74%) of those people infected by cancer were complaining from viral hepatitis. The owner of a weak liver is more exposed to primary hepatic cancer. One of the studies showed that the rate of infection by hepatic cancer between males was higher than it was with females by (6) times. And this is the result of menstruation, that "Divine Cupping".

Studies have shown that the tumor cells in the blood circulation, which saved them-selves from damage, become a malignant dissemination whose rate did not exceed one cell out of ten thousand cells from the total tumor cells because the effect of immunity was strong in the blood medium.

For this reason doctors started using anticoagulins to stop the spreading of the cancerous cells. Cupping heightens the efficiency of the immunity system in general and saves us from the trouble, the spoiled corpuscles the blood impurities. It reduces the blood viscosity, and raises its liquidity in a normal way without artificial induction, and the induction of bone marrows to produce more immunity cells.

This is what the lab studies have proved and were affirmed by our lab team. The spleen concentrates itself to practice its immunity role, and the systems of the body are rehabilitated, and heightened their capacities by cupping operation and in improving the patient's situation to a certain recovery of this malignant disease.

The cupping operation improves the eyesight resulting from insufficiency of perfusion and lessen clotting of blood by removing the extra congestive blood and eventually it lessens brain clots, and in reducing arterial pressure, it lessens occurrence of brain hemorrhage, and in strengthening immunity, it also lessens occurrence of neuro-immunity lesions. Without any doubt, science will discover other advantages for cupping in advance of time to show that it is an excellent helpful device in treating a number of diseases.

§§§§§§§§§

Chapter Six

- **The Simple Cupping Instruments**
- **The Mechanism of the Cup of Cupping (Known as air-cups)**
- **Application Method of the Cupping treatment**

The Simple Cupping Instruments

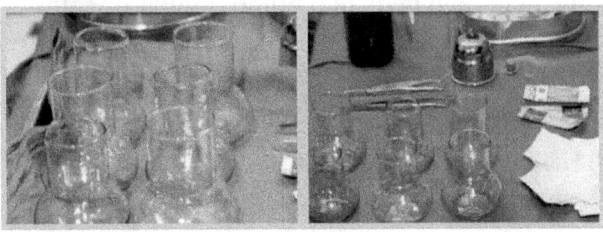

4- The cups of cupping are known as (air-cups).

They are simple glass cups, and they are available in the markets.

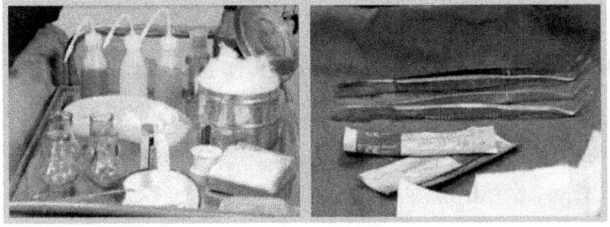

- Medical antiseptics for superficial cuts.
- A candle.
- Inflammable small cones of paper.
- Sterilized medical hand gloves.
- Sterilized medical scalpels.
- A pack of cotton and sterilized medical gauze.

The Mechanism of the Cup of Cupping (Known as air-cups)

Cupping tends to make a kind of blood congestion in the upper part of the back (the shoulder blades) by using special cups known as (air-cups) with a small potbelly and a little elongated neck of a diameter less than the belly and ends in a round regular opening.

In ancient times these cups were made from hollow horns of some animals or from the reeds of hard hollow plants such as the branches of bamboo (known to the Chinese). Then they were developed later to be made of hand-made glass because of easiness in cleaning and sterilizing and for its transparency which permits the cupping-practitioner to see the blood extracted from the cupped person.

We start burning a piece of paper made in a form of a cone, i.e. in the shape of a funnel. The piece of paper is better to be cut from a newspaper for easiness of burning and the possibility of inserting it through the opening of the used cup.

After inserting the burning cone into the cup, we stick the opening of the cup right away near the lower end of the shoulder blade (the scapula) in the place between the spine and the inside limit of the scapula. In turn, the burning paper will burn a big quantity of the air inside the cup and decrease the pressure, and hence it sucks the skin and pulls it out from the opening of the cup to equalize the decrease in pressure inside it, and as a result the local blood congestion takes place.

The pull on the skin and the little high temperature inside the cup cause a superficial vascular dilation in the region of the shoulder blade on which the cup is fixed. Also the blood succumbs to the pull and increases the redness of the place. Letting the cup pull the skin for a while (2-3 min) prevents the assembled blood from mixing with the circulation to a certain degree. After that the cupping-practitioner starts scratching some superficial cuts on the congested region of the skin (after removing the cup) by the edge of a sharp sterile blade taking into consideration the other complete practical rules of cupping in view of timing, age and the physiological condition of the body as we have already indicated.

Application Method of the Cupping treatment

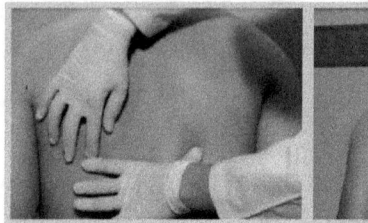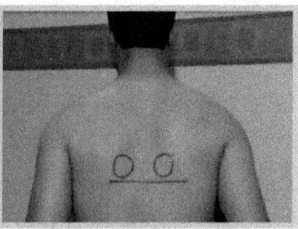

The cupping- practitioner prepares the papers clips and wraps them in the form of funnel cones taken from newspaper for easiness of burning. And in the morning of the day of cupping application:

The wishful person in cupping takes off his upper clothes and keeps his back naked after warming the room with a stove in order to make the surroundings warm (if it is not already warm). It is better to provide moderate warmth rather than hotness.

The person sits cross-legged, or sits in the way he could rest his body. Any way, he must sit somehow straight up. The practitioner lights a candle and fixes it near him. Then he puts on sterile medical gloves on his hands to start work

1) After sterilizing the skin region very well, the practitioner holds one cup in his right hand and the other hand holds a small conical paper and lights it from the candle. When the piece of paper burns well. He inserts it quickly inside the cup, and fixes the cup

quickly and lightly on the back in the two places, the right one and the left one, which we have already defined.

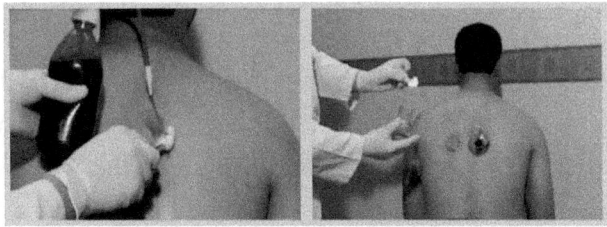

(The work requires lightness and quickness of hand which the practitioner acquires by practice. The operation is easy and facile).

2) Then he holds another cup and in the same way he fixes it in a symmetrical place of the first one. He must be sure of the fixing force of two cups on the body and their pulling force on the skin.

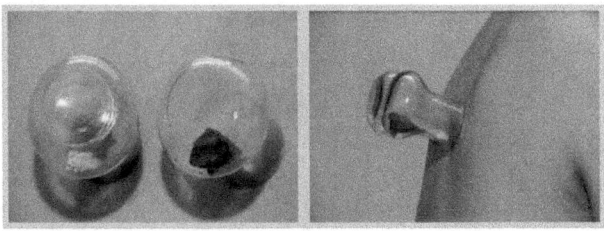

If the two cups are not strongly fixed, the practitioner must take off the weak cup and empty it from the ash and the rest of the burned cone, and then he repeats the procedure by burning another cone of paper, puts it inside the cup while it is at its utmost burning and fixing the cup on the same place.

Important Remarks:

- If there is hair on the back (the cupping place) of the person, the cupping-performer must only shave it with a razor in the limited symmetrical places for the two cups in order to fix them firmly on the body. Otherwise their adhesion with the skin will not be complete, the air can infiltrate into the cups and the adhesive force of both cups fails.

- The practitioner must keep the burning cone away from the opening of the cup lest it becomes hot and, in turn, it burns the skin a little on fixing it. When the practitioner repeats the fixation or refrains from doing it due to a weak fixation, he must change the cup with another one because the defect may be from the cup itself (due to a crack in it, or its edge is not regular, so the air gets through the cup). The most important thing is that the pull of both cups must be strong enough in order to get the best use of cupping.

- The practitioner must wait for (2-3) minutes letting the two cups to fix themselves on the back of the person. Then he takes off the first cup and empties it from the remains of the burned cone of paper and repeats fixing it by burning another paper cone. Likewise, he takes off the other cup, after fixing the first one, and re-fixes it as quickly as possible in order to prevent the congested blood from going away.

Remark:

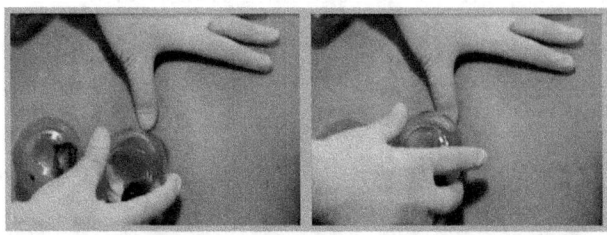

- For removing the cup from the body, we always resort to holding it by putting its belly between the thumb and the forefinger of one hand and at the same time by putting the other one on the body of the person on the upper part of his back adjacent to the mouth of the cup, and we press it on the skin while the holding hand pulls the cup downward from its belly by removing the upper edge and keeping the lower edge stuck on the body. When we remove the upper edge, the air fills in the cup and eventually we can easily remove the cup and put it away from the body of the person.

3) After the elapse of (2 - 3 minutes), we repeat removing the two cups and fixing them again (and these repetitions (twice) are made in order not to let the pull weaken in time).

4) During the last fixation (the last one) of the cups (in case the practitioner finds that the fixation of the two cups is weak and he cannot strengthen them, he repeats

the fixation for a fourth time). He starts in sterilizing the blade very well, or it may already be sterilized, and puts it in a piece of cotton wetted with antiseptic solution right from the beginning of his work.

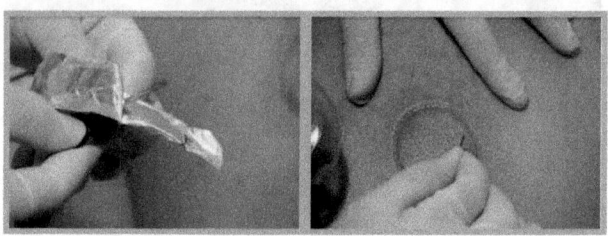

5) Then he lightly and quickly removes the first cup and disinfects its place with antiseptics or with sterilizing spray, and holds the angle of the blade in his hand, between the thumb and the forefinger, and slits the skin in superficial slashes apart (0.5 – 1 cm) from each other. He cuts few slashes up and down mentioning the name of God from the beginning of his work

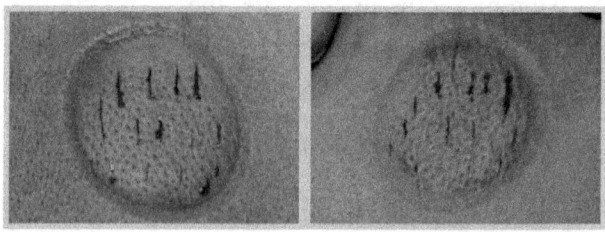

6) When he finishes the slight slashes in the first place, he fixes the cup on it slightly and quickly. Then the cup starts sucking the spoiled blood. The practitioner removes the second cup, disinfects its place and repeats the act of slashing and re-fixes it in the former place.

Important Remark

- The blade is to be used for one person exclusively, and then it should be thrown away in the wastebasket. It must never be used for another person even if it is disinfected with antiseptics.

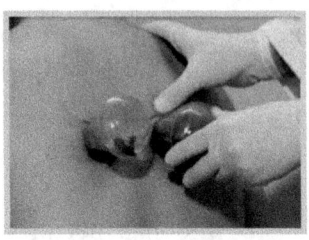

- The method of removing the cup is already explained by putting the potbelly between the thumb and the forefinger of one hand, and the other hand presses on the skin above the opening of the cup. Then the upper part of the opening is removed and the lower part of the cup is still stuck to the skin. Then the lower part is removed in passing it on the surface of the slashed spots and filling it with the withdrawn blood lest it runs down the back of the person. The slashed spots must not be dried with a soft paper-handkerchief or with a piece of cotton. The same cup must be re-fixed directly by burning a cone of paper.

- The person may be sufficed for four cups (two cups from the right side and two cups from the left side of the shoulder blades) unless he is suffering from strong diseases (except for anemia and blood depression). The practitioner may take two other cups so that the total amounts to six cups from the back of the person.

- The quantity of spoiled blood which is extracted for the first time by means of a medical cupping operation amounts to (100 – 200) grams while the quantity of a donated blood may amount to (450) grams. Therefore, the cupping-operation with its active magical cure is actually the cheapest price for harmful blood.

- He who has performed cupping in past years, will have no harm if he bleeds six cups in general or eight ones as most limit, especially for those who suffer from diseases as: Blood clot, arteriosclerosis, cancer, blood hypertension, arthritis, migraine, headaches in general, lumbago, pulmonary infiltration, cardiac infarction, angina pectoris, Diabetes, ischemia, paralysis, excess level of iron or Hemoglobin, hemophilia, downfall In heartbeats, cardiomyopathy, general neural diseases, leukemia.

- In respect with longevous people of weak stature, especially women, it will be enough to extract two cups utmost from every side even for those who are used to perform cupping every year unless cupping has exceeded in usefulness and the person insists on performing more so long as there is no harm, no obstacle.

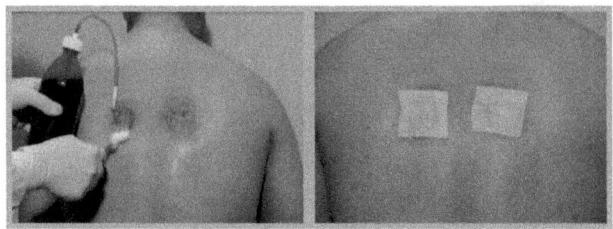

7) When the practitioner removes the last two cups, he must disinfect their places (the slight cuts) very well, and must put a piece of sterilized gauze sprinkled with a disinfectant solution by means of an atomizer on place of the cuts.

8) After the cupping operation, the person can eat a dish of "fat'toush" the ingredients of which and its way of preparation have already been explained, or he may eat a meal of vegetable salad.

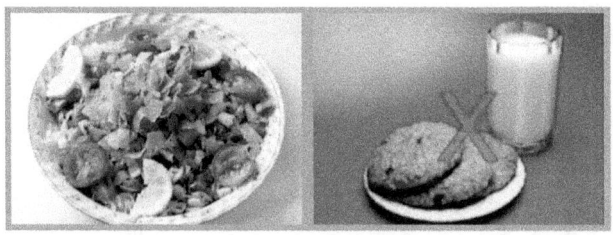

9) I want to recapitulate in here: it is forbidden for the cupped-person to drink milk[9] or eat any dairy products

---

[9] It is forbidden for the cupped-person to drink milk or eat any dairy products such as cheese, yogurt and cream, or eat any meal cooked in these kinds of dairy products during the day of cupping, i.e. only the day of cupping and its night because milk and its derivatives mostly lead to nausea and evoke vomiting, and make

all the day and its night only (for twenty-four hours) in which he has performed the cupping operation because milk contains calcium and some amino acids which lead to disturbances in blood pressure.

10) The cups must be cleaned and disinfected very well soon after the operation if possible, or they must be destroyed completely in a special place for rubbish.

---

disturbances in blood pressure; all that may lead to harm and some health problems

Chapter Seven

- **The general lab report of the systematic scientific study about the cupping operation**

- **Clinical medical research team**

- **Beware of the Conjurers and of those Panting for Money!**

The general lab report of the systematic scientific study about the cupping operation

In 2001 "prepared under the supervision of Dr. M. Nabeel Al-Shareef, the prior dean of the faculty of Pharmacy"

The study was preformed according to the scientific rules which the great Humane Scholar Mohammad Amin Sheikho deduced from the noble prophetic traditions. These rules state that cupping should be applied:

1) In the early morning, on fasting.

2) In the springtime, during the second half of the lunar months corresponding to April and May (in the Mediterranean countries as Syria).

3) For men over twenty years old, and for women over menopause.

The research included 300 cases which have been studied by a laboratory medical team and a clinical medical team.

The findings of the study came as follows:

1. In cases of hypertension, the blood pressure decreased to its normal limit.

2. In cases of hypotension, the blood pressure increased to its normal limit.

3. The electrocardiograms showed a great improvement, and graphically there was a return to normal situation in the segments slide.

4. Decrease to normal limits in ESR.

5. Moderation in the red corpuscles count.

6. In all cases of polycythemia (Erythremia), the value of hemoglobin decreased to its normal limit.

7. In all cases of low hemoglobin, its value increased to the normal limit. This denotes an activity in the body and a growth in its ability in producing benign young red corpuscles which help in more active and effective transporting of oxygen.

8. In 60% of the cases (cupped persons), there was a rise in leukocytes count within normal limits.

9. The count of leukocytes increased in 71,4% of cases of rheumatic diseases. This explains the instant recovery of the rheumatic patients and those who suffer from chronic inflammations after they use cupping.

10. Neutrophils count increased within normal limits in 100% of cases of rheumatic diseases.

11. In 83,3% of cases of asthma, the neutrophils count increased within normal limits.

12. Neutrophils count fall to normal limits in all cases of abnormal neutrophilia.

13. In cases of heart diseases, the neutrophils count fell to normal limits in the rate of 76,9% of the cases.

14. Rise in thrombocytes count in 50,6% of the cases.

15. In all cases of thrombocytopenia, the count of thrombocytes became normal.

16. In 50% of cases of essential thrombocytosis, the count decreased to normal limits.

17. Glucose level in blood decreased in 83,75 % of the cases, while it remained within its normal limits in the rest.

18. 92,5 % of cases of diabetic patients showed a decrease in glucose value.

19. Creatinine value in blood decreased in 66,66 % of the cases.

20. The quantity of creatinine contained in the cupping blood was high in all cases.

21. 78,57% of patients having a high level of creatinine in blood showed decrease in it.

22. The value of uric acid in blood fell in 66,66 % of the cases.

23. The level of uric acid in blood decreased, at the patients suffering from its rise, in 73,68 % of the cases.

24. The value of urea in blood decreased in 50,7 % of the cases.

25. Urea level in blood decreased in 80% of cases having a rise in it.

26. 80% of cases of high level of the liver Enzyme (SGPT) showed falling in it. This indicates that the liver has been activated after performing cupping

27. SGOT (a liver Enzyme) became lower in 80% of cases of patients having a high level of it. This explains the improvement that the electrocardiogram showed.

28. Alkaline phosphatase (a liver enzyme) decreased in 62,85 % of the cases where it was high.

29. The amylase level in blood became lower in 54,9 % of the cases.

30. In all cases of a high value of albumin in blood, the value returned to its normal limit.

31. The cholesterol level in blood became lower in 81,9 % of the cases.

32. Regarding the patients who had a high value of cholesterol in blood, the value decreased in 83,6 % of the cases.

33. The triglycerides level decreased in 75 % of the cases where it was high.

34. (K) and (Na) ions became normal in 90 % of the cases.

35. (Ca) ions became normal in 90 % of the cases.

36. /CPK/ decreased in 66,66 % of the cases where it was high.

37. The red blood cells in the cupping blood withdrawn from the upper part of the back were all of abnormal shapes: Hypochromasia – Burr – Target – Crenated – Spherocytes – Poikilocytes – Anisocytosis – Shistocytes – Teardrop cells – Acanthocytes.

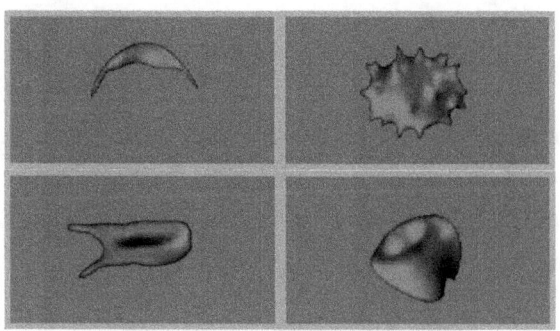

5- Some shapes of the red blood cells in the cupping blood

38. The leukocytes count in the cupping blood did not come to one tenth of their count in the venous blood. This indicates that the cupping operation keeps the components of immunity system in the body.

39. In 66% of the cases, there was an increase in the iron level within its normal limits.

40. (T.I.B.C.) was very high in the cupping blood where it varied between (422) and (1057) while in the venous blood it ranges between (250) to (400). This indicates that there is a mechanism which prevents iron from getting out of the cupping scratches retaining it inside the body so as to take part in building new blood cells. This is possibly associated with an activity in the process of iron absorption in the intestines.

41. (CPK) became normal in 92,4 % of the cases.

42. (LDH) became normal in 93,75 % of the cases.

These extremely dazzling findings reflected too many cases of marvelous recovery which came as a proof of the grandeur of the prophetic science and the weighty wonderwork brought by the first teacher our master Mohammad (cpth) and transported to us by the great humane scholar Mohammad Amin Sheikho.

"In the name of God, the compassionate, the compassioner"

A systematic study on cupping operation, year 2000 directed by:

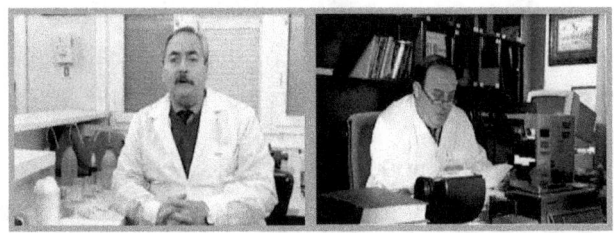

6- Prof. Dr. Mohammad Nabeel Al-Shareef (left) and Prof. Dr. Fayez al-Hakeem (right)

- Prof. Dr. Mohammad Nabeel Al-Shareef

- Prof. Dr. Fayez al-Hakeem

- Prof. Dr. Mohammad Mahjoub Jeiroudi

- Prof. Dr. Sa'ed Mokhless Yakoob

- Prof. Dr. Ahmad Samir Al-Nuri

- Dr. Mohammad Fuad Al-Jabassini

Our laboratory performed a blood-study on (330) cupped persons, and the findings were as follows:

First:

Cupping operation applied according to the correct scientific rules which are:

Cupping applied on men who are over the age of 20 years, in the early morning, on fasting, in spring, during the second half of the month of the lunar calendar and on the upper part of body back, we found:

1) Moderating of blood pressure and heart-pulse: where they became normal after applying cupping in all cases. This lessens the big loads tiring the heart.

2) The blood sugar level decreased in diabetic patients in a concentration of 39% of its high concentration (level) after cupping.

3) Rise in number of red corpuscles – within normal limits – in 33% of the cases, and remained within normal limits in the rest cases. This proves the effect of cupping in activating the marrow.

4) The shapes of red corpuscles in the cupping blood were always abnormal in all the cases:

- Hypochromasia.
- Burr cells.
- Target cells.
- Crenated cells.

Note: the blood samples were taken directly from the wounds before putting the cupping cups lest their low pressure may affect the shapes of the blood corpuscles.

5) Rise in number of leucocytes in 60% of the cases. This indicates that cupping operation stimulates the bone marrow for generating new corpuscles. The rate of rising is 10-15%

6) A very small number of leucocytes in the cupping blood in all cases of study. It varies only between 525-950 corpuscles/mm^3.

This requires a developed study to reveal the behavior of leucocytes in non-exiting with the cupping blood and consequently, the mechanism by which cupping operation keeps the components of immunity system.

7) Fall in the count of neutrophils in the cupping blood.

8) Rise in the percentage of lymphocytes (52-88%) in the cupping blood in all cases, while in normal case it should not exceed 35%.

9) Moderate level of iron ions in blood. It turns to the normal limits (60-150) if there is a rise or fall in it. Rising of iron ions rate to the normal limits in blood may be ascribed to improving its absorption in the intestines.

10) Very high rate of T.I.B.C. in the cupping blood. It varies between 250 to 400 in normal blood. This evokes

many inquiries and question marks?? How did the Iron-transferor (which has protein construction) get out with the cupping blood after it had unloaded its iron which remained in the body to partake of forming new blood corpuscles??

That is what we hope to be studied in the near future in order to recognize this unique mechanism.

11) T.I.B.C. was normalized within normal limits in all cases after cupping.

12) The level of triglycerides in blood was lowered in 83% of cases having high one of it, and it was normalized in the other of cases.

13) The value of cholesterol in blood was lowered, in patients suffering of its high level in, 70% of the cases.

This indicates an activity of liver cells so the liver performs its functions as metabolizing and discharging the surplus cholesterol and triglycerides perfectly.

14) The value of uric acid decreased to its normal limits in blood after cupping.

15) The platelets count increased – within the normal limits – in the venous blood after cupping.

16) Moderating of values of (SGOT-SGPT) in the venous blood after cupping.

17) High value of creatinine in the cupping blood while it becomes low one –within normal limits – in the venous blood after cupping.

18) Moderate level of blood ions (Ca – K – Na) in the venous blood after cupping.

Note: the rate of plasma in the cupping blood was less than 20%, while the rate of the other components was more than 80%. This reflects well on blood circulation in the body and lessens the chance of forming clots.

Note: the cupping blood coagulated despite putting it in tubes containing anti-coagulation (K3EDTA). This indicates that the cupping blood is abnormal.

§§§§§§§§§

Second:

Tests on cupping operation in conditions violating its precise scientific rules:

Tests on cupping under the stated age:
The studies proved that there is a big difference between the cupping blood taken from cupped-people over twenty years old (which is the suitable age for cupping) and that of people under this age. The results showed big similarity between the later blood and the normal venous blood in the count of erythrocytes and leukocytes and the normal shapes of the red corpuscles, as well as in the uric acid, the triglycerides and cholesterol.

This proves the falsehood of any saying calling to perform cupping on people under twenty years old. But the right condition is over this age, because the physical growth of man stops, therefore he needs cupping.

Tests on cupping after breakfast:
The cupping blood in this case seemed to be almost similar to the venous blood concerning the blood cells general count, the blood smear, and the normal shapes of the red corpuscles in both of them.

This affirms that the cupping operation should be applied only before breakfast in the morning.

Having food activates the blood circulation so as to help in digesting it and transporting the aliments to all parts in the body. This leads to carry awaying the blood sediments (aged, dead and tear red blood cells and other unwanted blood materials) which have settled temporarily between the scapulae during the night (sleeping).

Tests on cupping applied on places other than the upper part of the back:

The medical team performed many cupping operations on different places of body such as the leg and over the jugular veins, but the tests of the blood coming out of the cupping scratches in these places showed that it was too similar to the venous blood concerning the blood cells general count, the blood smear, and the normal shapes of the red corpuscles in both of them. Thus we can say that there is no substitute for the cupping on the upper part of the back (the true place of cupping on body).

Tests on cupping out of its regular time:

When performing the cupping operation at times other than its suitable one (that, in times other than the days of April and May corresponding to the second half of the Lunar month) and after making analytic studies on the blood of this cupping, the medical team found that the blood taken from this cupping have specifications similar to those of the venous blood concerning the blood cells general count, the blood smear, and the normal shapes of the red corpuscles in both of them.

This definitely indicates that any cupping operation is performed out of its defined time will avail nothing".

§§§§§§§§§

Clinical medical research team

General Supervisor on the Scientific Researches on cupping medicine: **Prof. A. k. John (alias Al-Dayrani)**

Members of the Clinical Medical Team:

Prof. Dr. Abdulghani Arafa
Specialist in Respiratory Diseases from Paris' University and Hospitals, Member of American Society of Pulmonary Diseases –Head of Syrian Society for TB treating and respiratory diseases.

Prof. Dr. Ahmad Takriti
Professor of Cardiac Surgery in the Faculty of Medicine – Damascus University – Specialist in Chest, the Blood vessels Surgery – Licensed (CES) and microscopic surgery from Paris.

Prof. Dr. Muhiddin Al-Saudi
Tumors Diagnostician and Therapist – PhD in treating Cancer Medicinally and Radiologically –Professor in Damascus University – Director Atomic Medicine Center in Damascus.

Prof. Dr. Abdulmalek Shalati
Neurologist from UK – Member of American Academy for – Head of Neurological Diseases department in Muwassa Hospital- Professor in Damascus University.

Prof. Dr. Akram Hajjar
Prof. in the Faculty of Medicine – Damascus University – Chief of head diseases Section – licensed by American Board body in ENT, Head and Neck Surgery.

Researcher Dr. Abdullatif Yassin
Specialist in Gynecological Surgery, Obstetrics & Sterility – M.R.C.O.G. in London – M.R.C.O. in Ireland – Obstetric & Gynecological Surgeon in London University, Hospitals.

Prof. Dr. Haytham Zoheir Al-Habal
Ophthalmologist and Eye Surgeon from London University, Hospitals – Head of Eye Section in Atomic Medicine Center – Supervising Physician in the Faculty of Medicine & Muwassa Hospital.

Prof. Dr. Amin Suleiman
Hematologist, Specialist in Blood Diseases & Bone Marrow transplanting from France universities – Professor of hematic diseases in Damascus University.

Prof. Dr. Marwan Al-Zahra
Specialist in Neuro-microscopic Surgery from UK – licensed by American Board body in Neurological Surgery from USA – Consultant in Neurological Surgery – Head of Neurological Surgery section in Tishreen Military Hospital.

Prof. Dr. Ahmad Ghiyath Jabakji

Specialist in Neuro-microscopic Surgery , Brain & Spinal Cord – Head Traumata, the Spine, Lumbago, Paralysis Diseases – Congenital Deformities – Head Traumata Certificate from Holland – Member of European Society for Nerve Surgery.

Prof. Dr. Abdullah Makki Al-Kuttani
PhD in General Surgery from Hannover University in Germany – Member of German Academy for Surgeons – Senior Consultant & Head of General Surgery, Surgery of the Digestive System & Its Tumors Section - Surgery of Hernias - Consultant in Medical speculum surgery from Germany

Prof. Dr. Ahmad Hassan Hawash
Specialist & State Licentiate in Diseases and Surgery of Blood Vessels and General Surgery from Charity Hospital in Germany.

Prof. Dr. Ahmad Afif Faour .
Specialist in Diseases and Teatment of Tumors – Head of Tumors section in New Ibn Rushd Hospital.

Prof. Dr. Riyadh Habboosh
Ophthalmologist, PhD in Eye Diseases and Surgery – Specialist in Glaucoma, Myopia Surgery and ocular lenses From Russian Medical Complex – Fiodorof - Lecturer Prof in Homs University.

Dr. Nabil Kamel Al-Salek

Specialist in Bone and Joint Surgery – F.R.C. S. from UK

Dr. Abdulaziz Al-Nahar
PhD in Obstetrics and Gynecology from Russia

And others

Members of the medical laboratory team

Prof. Dr. Mohammad Nabil Al-Sharif
PhD in Pharmaceutical Sciences – specialist in Pharmaceutical analytic Chemistry – Toxic, Food and Industry Analysis From Brussels – EX-Dean of the Faculty of Pharmacy – Professor in Damascus University.

Prof. Dr. Ahmad Samir Al-Nuri
Professor of Pharmaceutical herbal Drugs and Medicinal Plants in Damascus University – Faculty of Pharmacy - Chairman of the Association of Pharmacists in Syria – Member of Parliament.

Prof. Dr. Mohammad Mahjoub Jeiroodi
Head of the Medical Laboratories section in Muwsssa Hospital

Dr. Mohammad Fu'ad Al-Jabassini
PhD in laboratorial Medicine from France

Prof. Dr. Fayez Al-Hakeem

Licensed by the American Board body in Anatomical Pathology

§§§§§§§§§

Beware of the Conjurers and of those Panting for Money!

We started right from the beginning to fight against those ignorant people for practicing conjuration and mixing it with confirmed medical scientific matters which were verified and performed by the humane eminent scholar Mohammad Amin Sheikho for these simple medical surgical operations (cupping) which was practiced within the modern medical procedures.

It was testified by the masters of medicine of this century about the deep-rooted civilization. But the astonishing not good matter is to hear about some careless persons who exploit the interest of people in cupping operation in these days to realize their materialistic goals, even if it was on the account of the health of the citizens neglecting the strict scientific rules of cupping.

§§§§§§§§§

To watch the learning & documentary films about "Cupping", please visit our website:
www.amin-sheikho.com
info@amin-sheikho.com

Chapter Eight

- **A Glimpse of the Life of the Eminent Scholar Mohammad Amin Sheikho**
- **A Glimpse of the Life of the Researcher & Islamic Scholar Prof. Abdul-Kadir John alias Al-Dayrani**
- **Issued to the Great Humane Eminent Scholar Mohammad Amin Sheikho (His soul has been sanctified by Al'lah)**

A Glimpse of the Life of the Eminent Scholar Mohammad Amin Sheikho

(His soul has been sanctified by Al'lah)

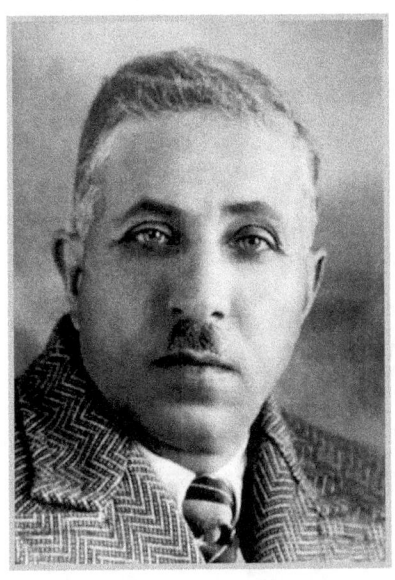

7- The humane scholar M. A. Sheikho

His honourable birth

His full moon appeared over Damascus in the year 1890 on a blessed night when a Damascene tradesman had a newborn baby. The father loved his son very much because he resembled the full moon in its beauty, and for his good clever presence.

In his childhood, he was active, clever, full of motion and cheerfulness so as to create a serenity and happiness of life in the hearts of those surrounding him.

Day by day he grew, and he showed an increase in cleverness and strength of personality, something which made his position greater before his parents. They venerated him and looked after him with love, affection and sympathy. But death soon snatched his affectionate father in his years of youth after an exhausting illness and tiring pain.

The death of the father had a great effect on the heart of everyone who knew him, for he left behind him a widow and two sons. Mr. Mohammad Amin had not reached seven years of age when he took responsibility for his mother's protection, defending her and keeping her away from the evils which appeared around his family after the departure of his father from this existence, and his older brother Saleem's travel to Turkey.

Even in his orphanage, Mohammad Amin was distinguished by his patience with the difficulties of life. He bore patience that mighty men could never bear, because he was an individual in a small respectable family that had faced many difficulties.

The sunrise of his youth & a glimpse of his deeds

Because of his honorable lineage that relates to the great messenger (cpth) he could approach the high responsible personalities of the ruling Turkish state at that time so that his family could reside in Sarouja Quarter which was called 'Little Istanbul', a dwelling place for the Turkish statesmen at that time. He also was able to study in the Royal Ottoman Faculty in Damascus, Amber.

He completed his studies when he became eighteen years old. He graduated in the rank of security officer. He surpassed his colleagues in extreme courage, trust, truth, hard work and his perseverance and continuous work with distinction. He headed many police-stations in Damascus and became director of its counties. He was the example, for no sooner had he taken his position than peace and safety prevailed in the region of his work.

He was the sleepless eye and the unmistakable arrow in the state's quiver. Whenever the state was confronted by a criminal or a crime, they used to ask for his help. When fear, killing, corruption and criminality spread over a region, he was the saving hope, who kept off danger and liberated people.

When decay began to bite the body of the Turkish state, and the torch of Islam was quenched, corruption and chaos prevailed all over the country until crime reached an unbearable limit, living became difficult, and the days were encompassed by danger, and the darkness of the night was horrifying: except in Damascus, its countryside and suburbs, for security was prevailing as a vigilant eye was watching and a merciful heart was dedicated to peace.

He faced storms of criminals in his work with courage and boldness, and he besieged many guerrillas and arrested their leaders. All his works were crowned in victory and support until he was surnamed 'Aslan', meaning 'the lion', for his audacity in facing difficulties. By his reliance upon God, he was the only officer who stood in the face of injustice and terrorism so that the criminals and thieves used to surrender to him, fearing his bravery, to offer a plea to his justice, mercy and contentment.

Thus he advanced in the ranks and was moved among the police-stations until he was appointed director of the citadel of Damascus, which contained the warehouses and the prisons. He remained in this position for a very long time during which he achieved glories and displayed bravery that Damascus had never seen before. He was very audacious in freeing thousands of prisoners with capital sentences and putting them in the front lines to defend the country against the infidel enemy. His action was the cause of removing the gallows which were planted by Jamal Pasha, the butcher, in the marketplaces and quarters of the country and which used to swallow hundreds of young men every day. For that reason he was exposed many times to death. Thus Al'lah saved him by His Greatness, His Mercy, and His Assistance.

During the French mandate, as he was a civil security officer, he was returned to his position as the director of a district or the chief of a police-station until the great Syrian revolution took place. Due to his love for God and his noble wish to serve his country, he was the iron arm of the revolutionaries and the aorta of the revolution. Its seal was in his trustworthy hand. He disquieted the French forces with his wonderful experiments in changing retreat into victory and in giving the revolutionaries the greatest arms deal between France and the Greater Syria. He handed these arms, which the French stored in Anjar castle in Lebanon, to the revolutionaries at night. General Catro, the governor of Syria at that time, lost his mind and ordered that Mr. Mohammad Amin be executed, but the Almighty God saved him and his assistant through His Complete Words, and he turned into a very trustworthy man for them despite their error of judgment.

The stage of guidance & invitation to Al'lah

After he became forty years old, God revealed to him His Omniscience.

He began to see the recitation of the prophet (cpth) in his prayer (communication with God) of 'Al-Fatiha' (the Opening) Fortress in sight and in hearing. After that he began to guide his disciples and he bore the banner of guidance in extreme strength and worthiness.

He used to be called 'Amin Bey' for 'Bey' is a Turkish word meaning 'the pure'. His salon used to embrace the flower of youth of Syria, Lebanon, and Iraq, asking for irrigation from his Mohammadan spring, rich and generous in giving an atmosphere of haughtiness, majesty, and sanctity.

If the noble deeds were mentioned...
In our horizons...
In you the example is given...
For all of us...

A glimpse of his invitation to Al'lah, his revelation and his great guidance

His sanctified assemblies were distinguished by charming and unique revelation in perfect and plain meanings, and complete presence of reality. His words used to hit the target and fall cool and peaceful in the hearts of the listeners, as a light that bewitched them to free their spirits to soar very high.

He drove away darkness, tore asunder contradictions, and finally obliterated the intriguing schools and barren argumentations which created a big gap in the minds of people between themselves and their God. He acquainted people with the reality of God, and the consummation of His Qualities... a Merciful God, Compassionate, Wise, Fair, Conferrer of benefit, Donator, deserved to be worshipped for Himself for He is the Owner of Beauty and Consummation. It is He who is praised for any harm because this harm results in cure and donation. He is Needless of creation, and of our allegiance and our obedience, because He is Rich and we are poor and our obedience is for our own good and benefit. We need to enter His luminous fort of faith, to be protected from misfortune and adversity.

His honorable life history was a high interpretation and a clear constitution for the wonderful revelation that he brought, which contained facts for which heads bowed. The reality was a light, the form was a proof and the true practical application was a guide. His revelation was matchless in world civilizations and the positive laws of present life.

- Why are we created?
- What is this universe for?
- What is the use of religious rituals?
- What is hunger for, followed by eating in Ramadan?
- What is the output and benefit of prayer?
- Why do pilgrimage to a waterless and treeless desert?
- Why were we brought into existence?
- Where were we?
- What is death for? And what is really after it?
- What is the spirit?
- What is the soul?
- What is the mind?
- What is paradise?
- What is hell?
- What about the problem of fate?
- What is the pre-material world (the world of spirits)?

Facts and questions have not come to people's minds because they were busy in the tempting world and its deceptions, and they forgot to search in the files of existence and know its secrets.

The famous coeval English scientist, Sir John Bennett, in one of his meetings with western scientists, said: "All the sciences that we have achieved are not equal to the sea of that great eminent scholar in the Orient."

His invitation to God is based on a course that is never mistaken: "Say: this is my way: I invite to Al'lah with sure insight, I and whosoever follows me. Glorified and Exalted is Al'lah. And I am not of the polytheists."

The Holy Qur'an,
Fortress 12, Yusuf (Joseph), verse 80

In the light of this honorable Ayah (verse), he began to call to God for more than thirty years a call concentrated on the following points:

Acquainting people with the consummation of the Almighty God, and showing His Mercy to His obedient people and His Justice with His creation. He refuted all that remained in human minds and whatever was circulated that contradicted the Godly Justice, Clemency, and Mercy and (all) Godly Consummations, and his guide was the Word of God: "And all the most Beautiful Names (Attributes) belong to Al'lah, so call on Him by them, and leave the company of those who deny His Names. They will be requited for what they used to do."

The Holy Qur'an,
Fortress 7, Al-A'raf (The Heights), verse 180

Revealing the consummations of the messengers (The Peace Through Them) of whom God witnessed in His Glorious Book as to their spirits' purity and their impeccability, and made them supreme examples for the worlds to be guided by them as mentioned in his book: The Impeccability of Prophets, – a book the like of which could never have been written by his forerunners. He confuted every fabrication or exegesis that disagreed with their sublimity and their high rank adhering in that to the Word of God "They are those whom Al'lah has guided, so follow their guidance…"

The Holy Qur'an
Fortress 6, Al-An'am (Livestock), verse 90

Calling people to adhere to honorable jurisprudence and to attain piety of God truly (witnessing by Al'lah's Light), besides warning people not to let their spirits follow their capricious whims, and not to depend upon vain wishes but turning to the Word of God: "It will not be in accordance with your desires, nor those of the people of the scripture; whosoever works evil, will have the recompense thereof, and he will not find any protector or helper besides God."

The Holy Qur'an,
Fortress 4, An-Nisa' (Women), verse 123

And also calling to the tradition of the messenger (cpth): "The discerning person is one who accuses himself and works for what is behind death, and the disabled is one who follows his caprices and asks God for wishes." "Narrated by Al-Turmozy"

Guiding people to the steps of true faith as shown by the messenger (cpth) to his noble companions, deriving them from the Book of God. No person has their heart mixed with delight of faith but they straighten for God's Order and have a self-deterrent (from committing sins). God mentioned that in His noble saying: "…and whosoever believes in God, He guides his heart."

The Holy Qur'an,
Fortress 64, At-Taghabun (The Apparent Loss), verse 11

Revering God's messenger (cpth), glorifying him, and showing his high position with Al'lah, then guiding to the way of his love (cpth) and revealing what fruit comes out of loving that pure chaste spirit, from entering into Al'lah's presence through him, and dying with a believing spirit coupled through him to perfection from God, following the Almighty's saying: "So those who believe in him, honour him, help him, and follow the light sent down with him, it is them who gain."

The Holy Qur'an,
Fortress 7, Al-A'raf (The Heights), verse 157

It was a valuable age that this pure man had spent striving and seeking nearness to Al'lah. And through this nearness he acquired the high ranks and consummation that he acquired, and realized glories and works charged with holy humane strife, and great humane sacrifices. So that his life was the highest example for the highest behavior, for supporting what is right through matchless heroic deeds that defeated falsehood and made it perishable.

He devoted his valuable life to the service of his human brethren. He competed with the wheel of time in its running and matched the sun in its light. The jet black nights of Damascus were changed at his hands into bright days for the glittering light of his works and the blessing grace of his sacrifices. He joined his night to his day overcoming rest. His eyelids never closed except for little naps to save his human brethren who were in swamps of sorrow and pain, not caring for the dangers of death or capital punishment or for what money or concessions he had paid in the service of God. Many times he remained penniless despite his previous wealth. It is no wonder that God revealed to him that manifest revelation on a sacred night to let him witness the realm of God and ascend in his spirit into the sacred lofty Mohammadan worlds which were prepared for him because of his truthfulness, effort and sacrifice. Similarly, anyone who strives to attain this and be truthful in their love and their quest for God and the messenger (cpth) shall find the door open for them and for every truthfully desiring follower.

Joining the Highest Comrade (his death)

In this wonderful way, he spent a valuable life full of knowledge of God, which the heart does not feel safe without, and without which humankind won't achieve happiness. He was the lamp that gave light to generations on their way to happiness through the Book of God, and the cresset that guided mankind to felicity, consummation, virtue and good life from God until he joined the highest Comrade in the first days of Rabi' Thani in the year 1964. He was buried in the cemetery of God's prophet 'Dhi Al-Kifl' in Al-Salhiyeh Quarter.

God says: "And who is better in speech than him who invites to Al'lah, and works righteous deeds, and proclaims: I am one of the Muslims."

The Holy Qur'an,
Fortress 41, Fussilat (Explained), verse 33

A Glimpse of the Life of the Researcher & Islamic Scholar Prof. Abdul-Kadir John alias Al-Dayrani

Verifier & Publisher of Books of the Humane Scholar Mohammad Amin Sheikho (His soul has been sanctified by Al'lah)

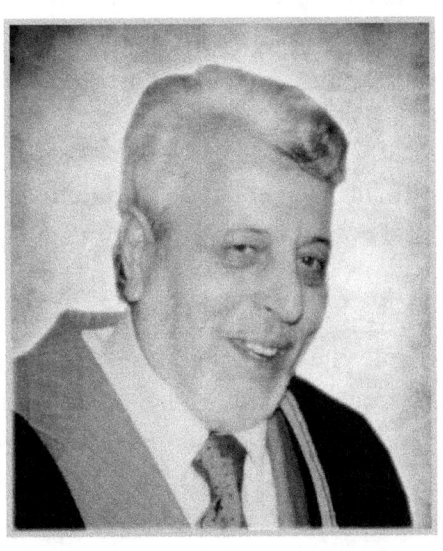

8- Prof A.K. John alias Al-Dayrani

His light rose on 24 July 1934, and he was lucky to see the light in the Damascene house of his father, a great scholar, Sheikh Mohammad Al-Dayrani (God has mercy upon him), a disciple of the great Sheikh Badrud-Deen Al-Hassani Al-Hussaini (God has mercy upon him), one of the great scholars of Hadith in Damascus at whose hands Professor Abdul-Kadir received a virtuous education full of knowledge. The extent of his learning was such that he left not one of his father's books unread in his youth.

Before he had completed his secondary education, he met with the scholar, M. A. Sheikho (his soul has been sanctified by Al'lah), and was astonished at his greatest of Godly sciences. He then adhered to him like his shadow for nine years, throughout which he was educated as a scholar. These were years full of great science and knowledge.

He finished his secondary education and started university, and got 10 university certificates.

Prof. Abdul-Kadir said:
These certificates have availed me no fact; rather, I got all the facts from my guide, the great scholar M. A. Sheikho. I have got a certificate in Arabic literature, but it has never profited me in philology or in understanding the meanings of language. I know the language with its meanings only from the scholar's mouth, and this is so concerning the other sciences.

All the books I have published are inclusively derived from the scholar's sciences, and include facts which have astonished every philosopher and scientist. Certain great sciences and witnessed facts are what I have received and heard from the great scholar's mouth; I have published them literally, as they are Godly revelations that cannot be attained by human science, even if all humanity assembled to aid one another. They are tangible and actual defiance, before which the sciences of humankind have vanished.

Some of these facts came to light and then removed obscurity; for example, the operation of cupping, which incomparably surpassed medicine when it cured diseases that had been considered incurable by the Arabic, Roman and Greek medical sciences for thousands of years. This has been noticed by millions of people who have applied cupping, and therefore, it is considered a miracle of the present age.

Similar to this is the secret of mentioning Al'lah's Name aloud over carcasses while slaughtering them, which was discovered by the great humane scholar and has been a mercy presented to the eaters of humanity and to all cattle slaughtered in this way.

In addition, there is what he presented in physics, such as discovering the sources of spring water, an issue which had not been known before by anyone.

Besides this are the great Qur'anic sciences, such as revealing the meanings of the letters with which the Fortresses start, and his wondrous explanation of the exordium (Al-Fatiha) and of the meanings folded under the verse: "Praise is to God, the Provider of the worlds"; and further, the meanings of each verse of the Holy Qur'an (Al'lah's saying). And there are other sciences of the scholar which contain facts which have not been discovered by anyone before or after him.

I hospitably accept any discussion about these sciences: a scientific impartial discussion far from emotions, seeking the truth and the absolute reality freed from any argument, quackery, or falseness.

Prof. Abdul-Kadir wrote a lot of collections through the Qur'anic lessons of his guide, the humane scholar, and he drank a lot from the spring of his sciences. He heard of the scholar's deeds from those who had witnessed them, just as he himself had viewed a lot of them.

When he devoted himself to guidance and the call to Al'lah, he collected, checked and examined what he had received from his scholar, and then he published these collections in order for their benefits to spread all over the world, in this time when humanity is greatly in need of such science.

The number of books which Prof. Abdul-Kadir Al-Dayrani has checked exceeds fifty-five, and his name has become widely known as being associated with the name of the great humane scholar M. A. Sheikho (his soul has been sanctified by Al'lah).

He undertook unique modern scientific research about the operation of cupping which the scholar had taught to his disciples from the right holy prophetic tradition, and he became the head of the Syrian medical team who carried out a modern scientific study of cupping, where all the requirements of research and the application of cupping rules were fulfilled under his auspices and with his guidance and consultation at every step. This study has been spread widely all over the world so that many Eastern and Western hospitals have seriously adopted it, and it has become the talk of people and their chief concern because of what astonishing cures have been achieved in this way.

He also did more scientific research to prove the wisdom behind mentioning the statement 'in the Name of God, Al'lah is Greater' aloud over cattle when slaughtering them.

This was an astounding modern medical method based on the tests of great scholars of medicine and through which it was confirmed that mentioning the Name of Al'lah results in purifying the cattle's meat from microbes, saving it from the pain of slaughter, and curing it from the incurable dangerous diseases like mad cow disease and bird plague. This was a subject which had been elucidated by scholar M. A. Sheikho (his soul has been sanctified by Al'lah) through giving his Qur'anic lessons to his disciples.

Damascus- on 4 Sept 2007

§§§§§§§§

Issued to the Great Humane Eminent Scholar Mohammad Amin Sheikho (His soul has been sanctified by Al'lah)

1) Interpretation of Am'ma Part of the Qur'an

2) Visiting the Prophet (cpth) and the Effect of his Love in Elevating the Believing Spirit

3) Impeccability of Prophets

4) High Schools of Al-Taqwa (Seeing by Al'lah's Light) – the Jewels of Rules in Explaining the Pillars of Islam

5) The Sources of Spring Water in the World

6) Interpretation of the Great Qur'an (Lights of Descending & Realities of Meaning) Volume –1–

7) Interpretation of the Great Qur'an (Lights of Descending & Realities of Meaning) Volume –2–

8) Am'ma Encyclopedia (The Compassionate's Gifts in Interpreting the Qur'an) Volume –1–

9) From the Heros' Careers for Children and Babies (The Courageous Boy and the Female Jinni)

10) From the Heros' Careers for Children and Babies (The Dog that Became a Horse) –2–

11) From the Heros' Careers for Children and Babies (The Brave Boy and his Practical Reply to His Uncle) – 3–

12) From the Heros' Careers for Children and Babies (Ring of Wrestling) –4–

13) From the Heros' Careers for Children and Babies (Disciplining the Greengrocer) –5–

14) From the Heros' Careers for Children and Babies (God Bless you, Cub of a Lion of the Quarter) –6–

15) From the Heros' Careers for Children and Babies (Adventure of the Little Horseman) –7–

16) Al-Amin Interpretation of the Great Qur'an (The Previous Nations) volume –1–

17) The Sources of Spring Water in the World – English translation

18) Pages from the Eternal Glory (the Life of the Great Humane Eminent Scholar Mohammad Amin Sheikho) Volume –1–

19) Reality of Intercession – A Calm Dialogue between Dr. Mostafa Mahmood & Dr. Yousef Al-Qaradhawi

20) The Reality of our Master Mohammad (cpth) Appears in the Twentieth Century

21) The Reality of our Master Mohammad (cpth) Appears in the Twentieth Century – Persian translation

22) Al'lah is Greater – Be kind to Animals: A Medical Scientific Study about the Use of Mentioning Al'lah's Name over the Carcass at Slaughtering

23) Islam… What is the Veil for? What is Divorce for? What is Polygamy for?

24) The West has Disenthralled Man from Slavery Why has Islam not?

25) The Great Scientific Discovery – the Astonishing Reality of the Six Days and the Seven Heavens

26) The Amazing Miracle of the Fundamental Verses of the Book in the Twenty-first Century

27) Faith – The First of High Grades of Al-Taqwa (Seeing by Al'lah's Light)

28) Prayer (Communication with Al'lah) – The Second of High Grades of Al-Taqwa (Seeing by Al'lah's Light)

29) Az-Zakat (Almsgiving) – The Third of High Grades of Al-Taqwa (Seeing by Al'lah's Light)

30) Fasting – The Fourth of High Grades of Al-Taqwa (Seeing by Al'lah's Light)

31) Pilgrimage (Hajj) – The Fifth of High Grades of Al-Taqwa (Seeing by Al'lah's Light)

32) A Calm Dialogue about the Great Humane Eminent Scholar Mohammad Amin Sheikho

33) Am'ma Encyclopedia 8 – Interpretation of Al-Ma'un (Almsgiving) Fortress

34) Am'ma Encyclopedia 9 – Interpretation of Quraish (All Creation) Fortress

35) Am'ma Encyclopedia 10 – Interpretation of Al-Fil (the Elephant) Fortress

36) Am'ma Encyclopedia 11 – Interpretation of Al-Humaza (The Traducer, The Gossipmonger) Fortress

37) Cupping: the Marvelous Medicine that Cured Heart Disease, Paralysis, Hemophilia, Migraine, Sterility and Cancer

38) The Great Humane Scholar Mohammad Amin Sheikho Retorts his Opposers

39) The Glorious Researches

40) The Mohammadan Revelations – (part 1)

41) Interpretation of the Great Qur'an (Light of Descending & Realities of Meaning) volume –3–

42) Unveiling the Secrets of Magic and Magicians

43) Al'lah is Greater – Be Kind to Animals – Persian translation

44) The Reality of Tamerlane the Great Appears in the Twenty-first Century – (parts 1 & 2)

45) The Second Coming of The Christ

46) Secrets of the Seven Praising Verses

47) Goodbye to Doctor of Al-Muqawqass

48) Contemplations on the Sciences of the Great Eminent Scholar M. A. Sheikho by Dr. Mustafa Mahmoud

49) The Second Coming of The Christ – English translation

THE END

Praise is to God, the Provider of the World

www.ingramcontent.com/pod-product-compliance
Lightning Source LLC
Chambersburg PA
CBHW051718170526
45167CB00002B/712